D1716645

Safety of
Diagnostic Ultrasound

PROGRESS IN OBSTETRIC AND GYNECOLOGICAL SONOGRAPHY SERIES

SERIES EDITOR: ASIM KURJAK

Safety of Diagnostic Ultrasound

Edited by

S. B. BARNETT and G. KOSSOFF

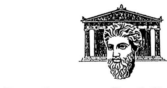

The Parthenon Publishing Group
International Publishers in Medicine, Science & Technology

NEW YORK   LONDON

Library of Congress Cataloging-in-Publication Data

Safety of diagnostic ultrasound/edited by Stanley B. Barnett and George Kossoff.

      p. cm.—(Progress in obstetric and gynecological sonography series)

   Includes bibliographical references and index.

   ISBN 1-85070-646-8

   1. Ultrasonics in obstetrics—Safety measures. 2. Generative organs, Female—Ultrasonic imaging—Safety measures. 3. Diagnosis, Ultrasonic—Safety measures. I. Barnett, Stanley B. II. Kossoff, George. III. Series.

RG527.5.U48S24   1997SS

618.2′07543—dc21

                               97-38076

                                   CIP

British Library Cataloguing in Publication Data

Safety of diagnostic ultrasound. — (Progress in obstetric and gynecological sonography series)

   1. Diagnosis, Ultrasonic—Safety measures

   I. Barnett, Stanley B. II. Kossoff, George

   616′.07543

   ISBN 1-85070-646-8

Published in the USA by
The Parthenon Publishing Group Inc.
One Blue Hill Plaza, PO Box 1564
Pearl River
New York 10965, USA

Published in the UK and Europe by
The Parthenon Publishing Group Limited
Casterton Hall, Carnforth
Lancs. LA6 2LA, UK

Copyright © 1998 Parthenon Publishing Group

First published 1998

Typeset by AMA Graphics Ltd., Preston, Lancashire, UK
Printed and bound by Butler & Tanner Ltd., Frome and London, UK

Contents

List of principal contributors   vii

Preface   ix

1   Introduction and overview   1
S. B. Barnett, G. Kossoff and D. A. Ellwood

2   Acoustic parameters used to describe diagnostic ultrasound exposure   3
G. Kossoff

3   Acoustic output of modern ultrasound equipment: is it increasing?   15
F. A. Duck and J. Henderson

4   Can diagnostic ultrasound heat tissue and cause biological effects?   27
S. B. Barnett

5   Effects of ultrasound exposure on fetal development in animal models   39
A. F. Tarantal

6   Sensitivity to diagnostic ultrasound in obstetrics   53
S. B. Barnett

7   Cavitation produced by diagnostic ultrasound pulses: can it occur *in vivo*?   63
C. K. Holland

8   Echo-contrast agents: what are the risks?   73
J. B. Fowlkes and E. Y. Hwang

9   Acoustic streaming and radiation pressure in diagnostic applications: what are the implications?   87
F. A. Duck

10   Studies of ultrasound safety in humans: clinical benefit vs. risk   99
J. P. Newnham

11   Cost-effectiveness of routine ultrasound in pregnancy   113
D. A. Ellwood

12   Regulations, recommendations and safety guidelines   121
S. B. Barnett and G. Kossoff

13   Take-home messages   133
G. Kossoff and S. B. Barnett

Index   141

List of principal contributors

S. B. Barnett
Acoustics and Ultrasonics Discipline
Division of Telecommunications and
    Industrial Physics, CSIRO
Bradfield Road
Lindfield 2070
Australia

F. A. Duck
Medical Physics Department, Royal United
    Hospital
Combe Park
Bath, BA1 3NG
UK

D. A. Ellwood
Department of Obstetrics and Gynaecology
The Canberra Hospital
Canberra Clinical School
University of Sydney
PO Box 11
Woden
ACT 2606
Australia

J. B. Fowlkes
Department of Radiology
University Hospital
Kresge 111, Rm 3315
Ann Arbor
MI 48109-0553
USA

C. K. Holland
Department of Radiology
University of Cincinnati, College of Medicine
234 Goodman Street
Cincinnati
OH 45208-0742
USA

G. Kossoff
Acoustics and Ultrasonics Discipline
Division of Telecommunications and
    Industrial Physics, CSIRO
Bradfield Road
Lindfield 2070
Australia

J. P. Newnham
University Department of Obstetrics and
    Gynaecology
King Edward Memorial Hospital for Women
Department of Obstetrics and Gynaecology
PO Box 134
Subiaco
WA 6008
Australia

A. F. Tarantal
California Regional Primate Research Center
University of California
Davis
CA 95616-8542
USA

Preface

This book was produced following encouragement by Professor A. Kurjak. We believe that it is an important element in the series *Progress in Obstetric and Gynecological Sonography*. It has the aim of promoting awareness and helping clinicians and research workers to keep abreast of current issues in the safety of obstetric ultrasound.

It has been our intention to produce a book that offers current information on aspects of the bioeffects and safety of diagnostic ultrasound that can be readily appreciated by a wide readership. We have made deliberate attempts to reduce the amount of technical jargon, whilst maintaining scientific reasoning and accuracy of detail. In that context, we have avoided creating a compendium of technical data and have almost eliminated mathematical and engineering formulae. The book is structured to present a logical progression of information from a description of the ultrasound output of modern equipment, through the types of biological effects that can be produced, to summaries of safety guidelines.

As editors, we recognize that writing chapters for books is an arduous task and we would like to express our appreciation to the authors who contributed chapters for this book.

Stanley B. Barnett
George Kossoff

Introduction and overview

1

S. B. Barnett, G. Kossoff and D. A. Ellwood

Since the introduction over 30 years ago of ultrasonic imaging as a diagnostic tool there has been an extraordinary growth in its clinical use. This has led to the development of a wide range of specialized procedures and the evolution of sophisticated modern equipment. Real-time imaging provides one of the greatest advantages of this modality. The frontiers of diagnostic medicine have been challenged by the ability to image the developing fetus, embryos and even the maturing follicles. Oocyte aspiration for *in vitro* fertilization procedures is often carried out under ultrasonographic visualization.

The use of ultrasound as an effective diagnostic modality continues to increase worldwide and equipment sales continue to exceed those of other diagnostic services. Improvements in resolution and image quality, and in gray-scale definition have been particularly important in obstetrics. Doppler measurement of fetal vascular hemodynamics is often used together with morphometric data to monitor intrauterine growth. The procedures have been further enhanced with the advent of endovaginal examinations, which allow direct access to anatomical structures without suffering the interference effects from overlying tissue that can occur in transabdominal examinations. The development of specialized applications such as color Doppler has provided the potential for further increasing the diagnostic effectiveness of ultrasonography.

These improvements in diagnostic ability have led to the development of sophisticated instrumentation that is very difficult to characterize in terms of acoustic output, because of the vast number of computations of exposure conditions that are adjusted by on-board computer software. It has become evident that there has been an associated trend towards increased power outputs such that modern equipment is capable of emitting acoustic power at levels that are sufficient to produce measurable effects in biological tissue. Knowledge of this has led to revision of regulatory standards by the Food and Drug Administration (FDA) Center for Devices and Radiological Health in the USA. There is also a more gradual process under way, through the International Electro-technical Commission (IEC), to establish internationally acceptable standards for the safe use of ultrasound in medicine. Slightly different approaches are being adopted, although the ultimate objective is similar: to put the responsibility of risk assessment in the hands of the operator. The FDA has taken a bold step and allowed relaxation of the output limits such that a substantial increase in the intensity may be applied to the fetus provided that the equipment incorporates an output display to alert the user to the relative risk of each examination. At the same time there is an increasing trend towards self-regulation whereby the ultrasonologist will ultimately decide on the risk/benefit ratio for each examination that they undertake.

In the past, the safety of diagnostic ultrasound was largely assumed on the basis of the absence of independently verified significant biological effects in mammalian tissue. A number of epidemiology studies had been reported, but these, generally, used gross morphological endpoints and often involved examinations in late pregnancy or well after organogenesis. The studies had many important limitations including small population size, often poorly matched controls, absence of information on acoustic output or even equipment type. The greatest limitation with epidemiology studies is that it is extremely difficult to find a positive association until the basic scientific research has established

1

a likely outcome, i.e. identified a testable hypothesis. The absence of reported bioeffects in humans at diagnostic levels does not necessarily mean that they do not exist, but rather that none has been detected that can be attributed with certainty to the ultrasound exposure. Only in recent years has it been recognized that the exposures from some new diagnostic applications might be capable of producing significant biological effects in tissue. This is due partly to reports of specific biological effects at relatively low intensities, and the growing awareness of the increased power emitted in some pulsed Doppler examinations.

Some fundamental issues have been questioned recently including both the risk to the fetus from ultrasound and the benefit to perinatal outcome of routine scans in pregnancy. In modern medicine the issue of cost-effectiveness of treatments is a matter of importance to the providers of medical specialties. The need for multiple ultrasound examinations must be justified on the basis of improved clinical outcome. If there is any doubt about the potential risk from such procedures then the justification should be much more thorough. It should be expected that referral for subsequent examinations is on the basis of the need to evaluate fetal growth and development and not because the initial examination was inconclusive. It must also be recognized that a real hazard of diagnostic ultrasound may be linked with inaccurate assessment. This should be considered as a potentially more serious issue than the consequences of some ultrasound-induced bioeffects. The potential for doing harm rather than good, from the patient's perspective, may stem from both inappropriate intervention and undue anxiety caused by either an inaccurate ultrasound assessment or careless reporting techniques. Whilst it is reassuring that there are few false-positive results in relation to fetal morphology scanning, inaccuracies in assessing gestational age, viability or even number of fetuses can cause major clinical problems. The impact of these on the patient, and on subsequent pregnancy outcome, needs to be studied in much more detail. Also, cost effectiveness of routine ultrasound use needs other factors to be taken into account which may have an impact on pregnancy outcome and subsequent infant development, such as earlier bonding and other positive effects on maternal behavior.

The developing international trend in diagnostic ultrasonography is for greater responsibility for risk assessment to be transferred to the user. The successful implementation of such changes requires a responsible attitude to education on the potential biological effects and in the understanding of the output display standards. The purpose of this book is to examine the current issues and concerns about the potential risk of biological effects and to provide advice, where possible, on the safety margins and relative risk of different diagnostic applications. It is important that users have an understanding of biophysics and bioeffects if they are to make informed decisions about the use of ultrasound and reduce the chances of causing bioeffects. Where there is uncertainty about the outcome or risk then it is appropriate to adopt an attitude of prudent use. In an assessment of the risk/benefit ratio one might expect the benefit to outweigh the risk in most cases where there is a real expectation of obtaining diagnostic data that would have an effect on the continuing medical management of the patient. The question of benefit of routine pulsed Doppler ultrasound in uncomplicated pregnancies is a matter of choice to be determined by national regulatory authorities.

Acoustic parameters used to describe diagnostic ultrasound exposure

2

G. Kossoff

SUMMARY

The transfer of responsibility to the sonologist to assess the risk/benefit ratio of an ultrasonic examination requires that the sonologist be familiar with issues of ultrasound exposimetry, in much the same way as the radiologist has an understanding of the physics of the dosimetry of ionizing radiation. The purpose of this chapter is to describe, in a non-technical manner, the acoustic parameters used to specify ultrasound exposure. Although the terminology is at first sight daunting, once the code used to describe the structure is appreciated, the terms become self-explanatory and descriptive of the features being quantified. All users of ultrasound need to develop this expertise to understand the significance of the acoustic parameters supplied by the manufacturers and to put into context the thermal and mechanical indices displayed on modern equipment as they relate to the assessment of the risk/benefit ratio of the ultrasonic examination.

INTRODUCTION

Diagnostic ultrasound is utilized in a number of ways to examine the fetus. For example, the transducer may be energized either continuously as in Doppler monitoring of fetal heart rate or pulsed as in ultrasonographic applications. The ultrasonic beam may either be stationary as in M-mode and pulsed Doppler examinations, or be scanned as in B-mode and color Doppler imaging. Finally, the transducer may be applied to the patient either transabdominally, over the perineum, or transrectally.

Despite the differences in these modes of application, the features of an ultrasonic field that are relevant to its ability to cause a potential bioeffect can be described by a small number of acoustic parameters of the field. The object of this chapter is to describe these parameters in a non-technical manner to demystify the terminology and to allow appreciation of the significance of these parameters in the description of ultrasound exposure.

PROPERTIES OF ULTRASONIC WAVES

Mode of propagation

Ultrasound is mechanical energy that propagates through tissue as an oscillating wave of alternating pressure. The elements of the tissue vibrate in response to the applied pressure and this forms the mechanism by which the ultrasonic energy interacts with tissue. The unit for pressure is a megapascal (MPa). As discussed in Chapter 3, diagnostic equipment is capable of generating peak pressures ranging from 0.5 to over 5 MPa. These are high values compared to the atmospheric pressure of 0.1 MPa.

The direction of vibration of the elements can be either along or at right angles to the direction of propagation of the ultrasonic wave. The former is known as a longitudinal wave, the latter as a shear wave. Liquids and soft tissue have resistance to compression but not to shear deformation. For this reason liquids and soft tissue support the propagation of the longitudinal wave only. Hard tissue such as bone can support the propagation of a longitudinal as well as a shear wave.

Velocity of propagation

The ultrasonic wave propagates through a medium with a velocity that is specific to the medium. For example, the velocity of propagation of the longitudinal wave in normal saline is 1540 m/s or 1 540 000 mm/s. The velocity of propagation in soft tissue is between 1 and 2% faster than in saline, while in fat it is about 10% slower. The velocity of propagation is a parameter that does not depend on frequency.

The velocity of propagation of the longitudinal wave in bone varies between 3000 and 3500 m/s, depending on the composition of the bone. The velocity of the shear wave is typically 20–30% slower than that of the longitudinal wave.

Wavelength

Wavelength is defined as the distance between two corresponding points on a wave. Wavelength is calculated by dividing the velocity of propagation by the frequency. For example, at 3 MHz, the wavelength in normal saline is

$$\frac{1540 \times 10^3}{3 \times 10^6} = 0.5 \text{ mm}$$

while at 5 MHz it is

$$\frac{1540 \times 10^3}{5 \times 10^6} = 0.3 \text{ mm}$$

Wavelength is of interest in diagnostic ultrasound because it determines the imaging resolution of the equipment. Typically the axial resolution of the equipment ranges between 2 and 4 wavelengths, while the lateral resolution ranges between 3 and 10 wavelengths. Thus at 3 MHz, the axial resolution ranges between 1 and 2 mm while the lateral resolution ranges between 1.5 and 5 mm, depending on the quality and cost of the equipment.

Attenuation

As the ultrasonic wave propagates through tissue, the energy content in the beam progres-

sively diminishes. Several mechanisms are responsible for this loss, and the term attenuation is used to describe loss of energy from all causes. Attenuation is frequently subdivided into (1) absorption, which involves loss/transfer of mechanical energy into heat; and (2) scattering, which involves loss/deviation of energy away from the main beam.

Body liquids do not significantly absorb or scatter ultrasonic energy and are generally considered to be non-attenuating. Their attenuation is, however, proportional to the square of the frequency and can become significant at frequencies above 10 MHz.

Soft tissue is a significant absorber but a relatively mild scatterer of the ultrasonic energy. Attenuation is proportional to frequency and is specified in terms of units of decibels (dB) per cm per MHz. For example, liver attenuates ultrasound at a rate of 0.45 dB/cm per MHz. Thus, a one-way propagation through 6 cm of liver tissue by a 5-MHz beam diminishes the energy content by

$$0.45 \times 6 \times 5 = 13.5 \text{ dB}$$

Bone is a significant absorber as well as a scatterer of energy in the longitudinal wave. Also, when energy impinges on bone at angles other than the normal angle of incidence, some of the energy is transformed into a shear wave, which is very rapidly attenuated by bone. For these reasons it is frequently assumed that all of the energy that penetrates bone is fully attenuated at the anterior surface of the bone.

Air-containing soft tissue such as lung absorbs as well as scatters ultrasonic energy. The attenuation is high and energy is dispersed throughout the tissue. As a consequence, air-containing lung is not amenable to examination by ultrasound.

Beamwidth

The ultrasonic wave emanates from the transducer in a beam-pattern that is determined by the dimensions of the transducer and the frequency. The beamwidth specifies the lateral dimensions of the beam-pattern. It is an important acoustic parameter in that it determines the lateral resolution of the diagnostic equipment.

It is also important in dosage considerations because all of the energy in the ultrasonic wave is contained within the beamwidth.

The beam-pattern generated by a single-element disk transducer consists initially of a cylindrical beam, the diameter of the beam being equal to the diameter of the transducer. The beam propagates in this form for a certain distance known as the near-field. The near-field is proportional to the square of the diameter of the transducer and inversely proportional to the frequency. Beyond the near-field, at distances known as the far-field, the beam changes into a cone and diverges at a constant angle which is proportional to the diameter of the transducer and inversely proportional to the frequency.

Focusing is used to narrow the beam so as to improve the lateral resolution. Unfortunately, it is not possible to narrow the beam over the total examination depth and a reduction in beamwidth is obtained only in the focal zone, typically over a distance corresponding to one-third of the examination depth. Diffraction considerations dictate that focusing can be achieved only in the near-field of the transducer.

Annular array transducers generate an axially symmetric beam and, as in the case of a single-element disk transducer, the beamwidth is simply the value of the diameter of this beam. Linear and phased array transducers generate a rectangular beam, and beamwidth has width and height dimensions.

High performance equipment employs dynamic focusing to improve the lateral resolution of the equipment during reception. Dynamic focusing does not change the shape of the transmitted beam and is not relevant in exposimetry considerations.

Pulsed mode of operation

The majority of ultrasonic diagnostic equipment functions in a pulsed mode[1]. The transducer is energized for only a short period of time and for most of the time it is used in receive mode collecting the sonographic data.

Figure 1 (a) illustrates a typical waveform used in B-mode and color Doppler imaging. The waveform is short, consisting of several cycles of the fundamental frequency of the transducer. Frequency is defined as the inverse of the duration of the largest cycle in the waveform. The waveform is characterized by a fast rise-time, the maximum pressure being reached by the first or second cycle, and a gradual decay, which lasts for a few cycles.

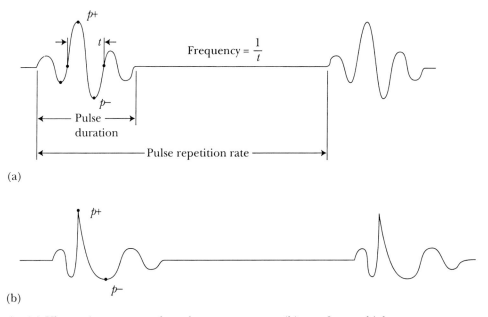

Figure 1   (a) Ultrasonic pressure pulse at low power output; (b) waveform at high power output

5

Pulse duration is generally given in units of microseconds (μs, or 10^{-6} s). The time interval between pulses is known as the pulse repetition period and, as it lasts longer, is generally given in units of milliseconds (ms or 10^{-3} s). The pulse repetition frequency and the duty ratio are two other commonly quoted parameters. The former is the inverse of the pulse repetition period and the latter is the ratio of the pulse repetition period over the pulse duration.

Non-linear properties of media

As the ultrasonic pressure wave propagates through a medium, the elements are subjected to a positive and a negative pressure. During the positive phase of the wave the elements are compressed, and during the negative phase they are pulled apart. This changes the density of the medium so that it is a little more dense during the positive phase and less dense during the negative phase of the pressure wave. The velocity of propagation of the ultrasonic wave changes with the density of the medium. Thus, the positive components of the wave propagate slightly faster than the negative components. At sufficiently high pressure, this effect can lead to a gradual distortion of the wave whereby the positive components of the wave bunch up, leading to the development of a steep positive wavefront, referred to as a shock wave[2]. The negative components also suffer some distortion and the negative portion of the wave is compressed and stretched out by a small amount.

The peak positive value of the pressure in the wave is known as the peak compressional ($p+$) pressure and the peak negative pressure as the peak rarefactional pressure ($p-$). In an undistorted wave these two values are equal. In a fully developed shock wave, as shown in Figure 1 (b), $p+$ can be up to three times greater than $p-$.

The physical properties of liquids are conducive to the formation of a shock wave. However, even in these media, a fully developed shock wave is observed only in the focal zone of a well focused transducer and at the high levels of output of modern equipment. The attenuating properties of tissue reduce the development of a shock wave and the effect does not develop

to a significant degree during propagation in tissue. This does not mean that the effect may be totally dismissed in exposure considerations. An example where it can be significant is in the propagation in the urine in the maternal bladder where the shock wave has opportunity to develop and the consequent transmission of this shock wave into the fetus lying posteriorly.

Power and intensity

Energy is defined as ability to do work. Work is done by the ultrasonic wave when the pressure of the wave acts against the resistance to deformation by the elements of the tissue to produce the vibration movements. If there is no resistance to the deformation, no work is done. Liquids conform to the shape of their containers and have little resistance to deformation. Thus little work is done and only a small amount of energy is lost as the ultrasonic wave propagates through liquids. Soft tissues hold their shape and it is this resistance to deformation which represents the mechanism for absorption losses manifested by tissues.

Power is defined as the rate at which energy is transformed from one form into another, such as from mechanical into thermal form:

$$\text{Power} = \frac{\text{energy}}{\text{time}}$$

Power is specified in watts, whereas energy is specified in joules. It is an important exposure parameter in that it is a major determinant of the ability of the ultrasonic beam to heat tissue.

Intensity is the spatial concentration of power:

$$\text{Intensity} = \frac{\text{power}}{\text{area}}$$

Intensity is specified in watts/square meter or some derivative there of, such as mW/cm^2. It turns out that intensity is proportional to the square of the pressure in the ultrasonic wave. Intensity can therefore be calculated if the pressure is known. Measurement of power and pressure is generally performed using different methodologies; the ability to derive intensity by two independent methods is useful in allowing a cross check on the accuracy of the measurements[3].

Intensity is a parameter that is space- and time-dependent. As such it is frequently misunderstood, misinterpreted or misapplied. The following illustrate three space-dependent definitions of intensity. The average intensity is defined as the intensity obtained by dividing the power by the area enclosed by the beamwidth. Close to the transducer, before the ultrasonic beam is able to form its shape, the beamwidth is equal to the physical dimensions of the transducer. The average intensity obtained by dividing the power by the surface area of the transducer accurately reflects the uniform intensity distribution across the beam at the surface of the transducer.

As one moves away from the transducer, the ultrasonic beam forms into the shape determined by the frequency and the physical dimensions of the transducer. The distribution of the energy across the beam becomes non-uniform and, as illustrated in Figure 2, there is concentration of energy on the axis. The average intensity obtained by dividing the power by the beamwidth grossly underestimates the axial intensity, typically by a factor of 3–5. As a bioeffect is most likely to occur where there is maximum intensity, the axial rather than the average intensity is the parameter of greater interest at distances away from the transducer.

The peak spatial intensity is the maximum intensity in the beam-pattern. In water it corresponds to the axial intensity at the focal distance. In tissue, because of attenuation, it may occur at a distance closer to the transducer.

The time-dependence of intensity is best illustrated by considering the ultrasonic pressure wave shown in Figure 1. Intensity is proportional to the square of the pressure; the time course of the intensity associated with that wave is shown in Figure 3. The square of a negative value is a positive number. Thus, the intensity in the wave has only positive values which range from zero to some peak temporal value. Indicated in Figure 3 are some of the temporal definitions for intensity. The spatial peak temporal peak intensity (I_{SPTP}) is the peak value of the intensity in the waveform. The maximum

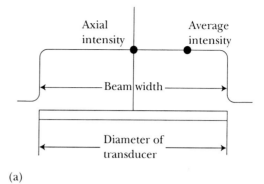

(a)

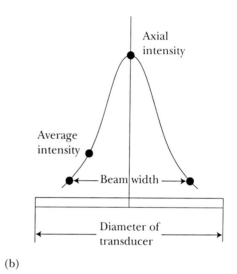

(b)

Figure 2 Intensity distribution (a) very near the transducer and (b) at the focus

intensity (I_m) is the intensity content in the largest single half-cycle in the waveform. The spatial peak pulse average intensity (I_{SPPA}) is the intensity content in the whole pulse, and the spatial peak temporal average intensity (I_{SPTA}) is the spatial peak pulse average intensity I_{SPPA} divided by the duty ratio. These terms are described in more detail in other publications on exposimetry[4].

Decibel notation

The decibel notation is frequently utilized in the description of ultrasonic exposure. It is a descriptor that compares the value of a parameter

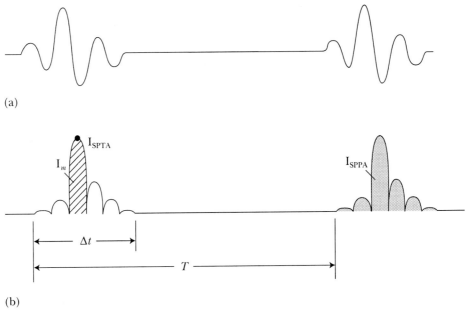

Figure 3 (a) Ultrasonic pressure pulse and (b) intensity waveform. I_{SPTA}, spatial peak temporal average intensity; I_{SPPA}, spatial peak pulse average intensity; I_m, maximum intensity. Duty ratio $= \dfrac{T}{\Delta t}$; $I_{SPTA} = I_{SPPA} \times \dfrac{\Delta t}{T}$

at the output to the value at the input. Examples of parameters of interest in ultrasound exposure include energy, power, intensity, pressure and voltage.

In the case of energy, power and intensity, the decibel (dB) is defined as ten times the logarithm of the ratio of the energy, power or intensity at the output to the energy, power or intensity at the input, i.e.:

$$dB = 10 \log \frac{energy_{output}}{energy_{input}}$$

In the case of pressure and voltage, the decibel is defined as 20 times the logarithm of the ratio of the pressure or voltage at the output to the pressure or voltage at the input:

$$dB = 20 \log \frac{pressure_{output}}{pressure_{input}}$$

Because energy, power and intensity are proportional to the square of the pressure or of the voltage, and as the logarithm of the square of a number is equal to twice the logarithm of the number, these two definitions for the decibel are in fact identical.

As ultrasound propagates through tissue there is gradual diminution of energy. The ratio of energy at output to energy at input is therefore less than one. The logarithm of a number less than one is a negative number. Attenuation by tissue is therefore specified by a negative decibel number, the negative sign indicating that there is loss of energy while the magnitude of the number indicates the amount of loss.

There are a number of advantages to the decibel notation which are based on the mathematical properties of logarithms. For example, if the ultrasonic energy propagates through two tissues with different attenuation, the total attenuation is obtained by simply adding the two decibel attenuation values.

Logarithms compress the magnitude of numbers. For example, the logarithm of 10 is 1, of 100 is 2, of 1000 is 3, etc. In the decibel notation, an energy loss by a factor of 10 is equivalent to −10 dB, of 100 to −20 dB, of 1000 to −30 dB, etc.

Table 1 lists some of the commonly encountered energy loss factors and the equivalent value of attenuation. Other values may be derived from those listed, using the relationship

Table 1 Energy loss factor and equivalent attenuation

Energy loss factor	Attenuation (dB)
1	0
1.3	−1
2	−3
4	−6
10	−10
100	−20
1000	−30

that the product of the two energy loss factors is the sum of the two attenuation values.

The following illustrates the ease of use of the decibel notation. Consider a case when propagation through tissue results in an energy loss by a factor of 16. This can be reduced to a loss of (4×4). From Table 1 this is equivalent to $-(6 + 6)$ dB, i.e. an attenuation of -12 dB. Consider a case when the attenuation is -36 dB. This can be reduced to $-(20 + 6 + 6 + 3 + 1)$ dB. From Table 1, this is equivalent to an energy loss of $(100 \times 4 \times 4 \times 2 \times 1.3)$, i.e. by a factor of 2080.

ACOUSTIC PARAMETERS USED TO DESCRIBE ULTRASOUND EXPOSURE

Over the years many acoustic parameters have been used to describe acoustic exposure. Initially, owing to limited availability of measuring equipment, only the power output or the average intensity was used to describe the exposure. An example of this approach was the early American Institute of Ultrasound in Medicine (AIUM) recommendation for an upper limit of 100 mW/cm^2 for the average intensity.

The development of miniature hydrophones gave investigators the ability to measure the ultrasonic pressure wave quantitatively and calculate the intensity in the various parts of the wave. This capability allowed, for example, the Food and Drug Administration regulatory authority in the USA to specify permissible levels of acoustic output for cardiac, vascular, ophthalmic and fetal applications[5] expressed in terms of three parameters for intensity, namely I_{SPTA}, I_{SPPA} and I_m.

With time, it was recognized that these three intensities did not allow adequate comparison of the ability of different ultrasonic beams to produce a potential bioeffect. The emphasis has since shifted to the use of parameters that more closely permit such comparison. This has resulted, for example, in the introduction by the AIUM of on-screen real-time display of non-acoustic indices such as the thermal and the mechanical index to describe the output being generated by the equipment. These indices, however, require measurement of the acoustic power output and of the maximum negative pressure $p-$ in the wave. An understanding of the significance of acoustic parameters still underpins the appreciation of issues involved in the description of ultrasound exposure.

Currently the acoustic output of diagnostic equipment is specified in terms of the maximum value of four acoustic parameters of the ultrasonic field. The first two parameters, the acoustic power output and the spatial peak temporal average intensity I_{SPTA}, relate to the ability of the ultrasonic beam to heat tissue and so potentially cause a thermally induced bioeffect. The third and fourth parameters, the spatial peak pulse average intensity I_{SPPA} and the peak negative pressure $p-$ describe the intensity content and peak pressure value of the transmitted pulse waveform and relate to the potential ability of the pulse to cause a cavitationally induced bioeffect.

It is recognized that the first two parameters do not permit calculation of the actual temperature rise in tissue. For this it is also necessary to know the value of other acoustic field parameters such as beamwidth and frequency, and of acoustic and physical properties of tissues such as attenuation and perfusion. Similarly, the last two parameters are insufficient to predict possible occurrence of cavitation in tissue. Indeed, the theory for cavitation in tissue has not as yet been formalized, and there are many uncertainties in our understanding of the requirements necessary for the development of cavitation in biological liquids and in soft tissue. Nevertheless, it is generally agreed that these four parameters allow a qualitative assessment and comparison of output of different equipment, and Chapter 3 describes the acoustic output of modern ultrasound equipment in terms of these parameters.

Acoustic power output

When an ultrasonic beam, propagating in water, impinges on an absorbing target such as a piece of butyl rubber, the target experiences a radiation pressure force that is proportional to the power contained in the beam. The radiation pressure force is relatively small; a beam with a power content of 1 W exerts on the target a weight of 0.067 g. As given in Chapter 3, the power output of modern equipment ranges from 1 to 500 mW, and is capable of generating a radiation pressure weight ranging from 0.067 to 0.0335 g. Although small, this radiation pressure weight can be measured by attaching a rubber target to the measurement arm of a sensitive analytical balance and noting the increase in weight of the target when the transducer is energized.

In M-mode and pulsed Doppler, the ultrasound beam is stationary and the size of the absorbing target needs to be just a little larger than the beamwidth to measure the energy content in the beam. In B-mode and color Doppler, the ultrasound beam is scanned to form the image. In this application the size of the target needs to be large, to ensure that all of the beams forming the image are intercepted and contribute to the power output measurement.

In a stationary beam all of the power propagates through the same tissue. A scanned beam insonates a large cross-section of tissue and, for the same power output, the power density per unit of tissue is reduced. This is relevant in the calculation of the potential temperature elevation in tissue. To allow this calculation, current standards also require specification of acoustic power output with a 1-cm blocking baffle placed in front of the absorbing target. This dimension is chosen to simulate the thermal perfusion characteristics of tissue; i.e. it is assumed that a temperature elevation 1 cm away from the point of interest is reduced by perfusion to have no effect on the temperature at that point.

Spatial peak temporal average intensity

The I_{SPTA} is measured by a calibrated hydrophone. These hydrophones are very small (typically 0.5 mm in diameter) transducers made from a piezoelectric plastic film. The sensitivity of these hydrophones compared to conventional transducers is low, but they have a very large bandwidth and are capable of accurately measuring the shape of the transmitted pulse. The hydrophones are calibrated by being placed in a known ultrasonic field and the magnitude of the received voltage measured. The calibration curves come with purchase of the hydrophone and can be trusted to remain stable for 2 years. It is good practice to have the hydrophones recalibrated beyond this period. They are delicate devices and require appropriate care during utilization to ensure that they maintain calibration.

In contrast to the large absorbing target that measures the acoustic power output of the whole beam, the point hydrophone samples only a small part of the ultrasonic beam. The hydrophone is therefore scanned around to ensure that it is positioned on the axis of the ultrasonic beam and at the focal distance from the transducer so as to measure the maximum spatial intensity.

A typical waveform received by a hydrophone is illustrated in Figure 1. The intensity waveform is obtained by squaring this waveform. The resultant waveform is shown in Figure 3. The spatial peak pulse average intensity is obtained by integrating this waveform, i.e. calculating the area under the waveform. Figure 3 shows that the ultrasonic pulse has a certain duration (t) and that the pulses are repeated every (T) seconds. The spatial peak temporal average intensity is obtained by multiplying the spatial peak pulse average intensity by the pulse duration (t) and dividing it by the pulse repetition time (T). Most well equipped laboratories have a small computer attached to the hydrophone to allow these calculations to be performed automatically.

The previous discussion described the calculation of the spatial peak temporal average intensity of a beam that is stationary, i.e. when the hydrophone measures the same axial intensity every repetition pulse. With a scanned beam, the hydrophone measures the axial intensity only once per image frame. The spatial peak temporal average intensity of a scanned beam is therefore obtained by dividing the value calculated for the stationary beam by the image frame rate, which typically is between 10 and 30 frames/s.

In order to have good lateral resolution, the beam is scanned in such a way that with each repetition pulse it moves across the focus a distance equal to about half the beamwidth. In this case, as illustrated in Figure 4, a hydrophone measures once every frame one maximum axial intensity value when the beam faces the hydrophone directly and two reduced values when the beam is directed on either side of the hydrophone. To avoid extra measurements, it is generally assumed that these reduced values are equal to half the value measured on the axis. The effect for beam overlap is therefore compensated for by multiplying the previously described calculation for spatial peak temporal average intensity by a factor of two.

All of these factors influence the value of the spatial peak temporal average intensity in the various equipment operating modes and is one of the reasons why this parameter covers the large range of values given in Chapter 3.

Spatial peak pulse average intensity

The I_{SPPA} illustrated in Figure 3 describes the intensity contained in each pulse. As discussed in the previous section it is a parameter that is required for the derivation of the spatial peak temporal average intensity. As the likelihood of

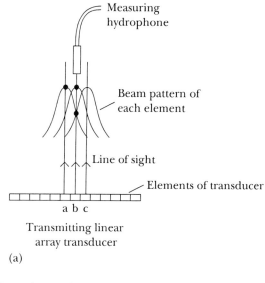

(a)

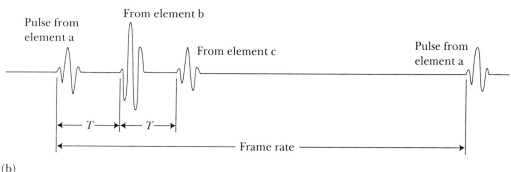

(b)

Figure 4   (a) Intensity measurement set-up; (b) signal received by hydrophone

the onset of cavitation is related to the spatial and temporal concentration in intensity, it is also used on its own merit as a descriptor for the potential of the ultrasound exposure to cause a cavitationally induced bioeffect.

As mentioned, there are many gaps in our knowledge of the requirements necessary for development of cavitation in biological media. As such knowledge is derived, it could well be that this parameter will be superseded or be complemented by other parameters which would be better reflections of the possible onset of cavitation in tissue.

Peak negative pressure

It is generally accepted that the peak pressure in the ultrasonic wave is an important determinant of the potential of the wave to initiate cavitation. At the high acoustic output generated by modern equipment the ultrasonic wave, propagating in water, undergoes a progressive distortion of the type illustrated in Figure 2. The wave becomes asymmetric, the positive component developing a steep shock front while the negative component incurs a stretching form of distortion. In a fully developed shock wave the peak positive pressure may be three times greater than the peak negative pressure. Accurate measurement of the fast rising shock wavefront is however, difficult and requires specialized calibration equipment.

The steep slope of the shock wave indicates that the wave contains beside the fundamental also many higher harmonic frequencies. It is not clear to what extent the development of shock waves occurs in soft tissue. These preferentially attenuate the higher frequencies, negating the development of the shock wave. Because of the difficulty in measuring the amplitude of the positive peak pressure accurately and the uncertainty in the degree of development of the shock wave in tissue, the current practice is to use the peak negative pressure as the descriptor of the peak pressure in the wave.

Water vs. *in situ* values

Measurement of acoustic parameters whether by an absorbing target or by a hydrophone is performed in a water tank. The values of the various parameters measured in this way are referred to as the water values.

Some authorities, particularly in the USA favor specification of *in situ* values of acoustic parameters. The rationale is that tissue attenuates the ultrasonic beam and the distribution of energy in an attenuating medium differs from that in water. For example, the value of the peak intensity at the focus can be significantly different, owing to attenuation of the energy on its way to the focus. Indeed, in media with an attenuation value typical of tissue the position of maximum intensity in tissue is closer to the transducer and differs significantly from that found in water.

The difficulty relates to the type of model used to simulate tissue and how well this model approximates the situation encountered in a patient. Several models have been proposed for a variety of applications: the average tissue model, where it is assumed that tissues attenuate the ultrasonic beam uniformly by 0.3 dB/cm per MHz; the bone model, where all of the energy is attenuated close to the transducer; and the first- and third-trimester models, where there is a non-attenuating water path between the transducer and the embryo/fetus. Other models to mimic applications such as transvaginal examinations are also in the process of development.

To date, the average tissue model has been the only model that has been used to give the value of acoustic parameters in specifications of acoustic output. These values are referred to as *in situ* values and, because of attenuation, are always less than the water values.

DISCUSSION

Considerations regarding possible harmful thermal and/or cavitational bioeffects impose overall restrictions on the range of values for acoustic parameters used by equipment functioning in the various modes used to examine the fetus. For example, thermal considerations dictate that, to avoid a significant temperature elevation, the total amount of acoustic energy should not be exceeded. The amount of temperature elevation is proportional to the product of the amplitude of the ultrasonic wave, the length of the ultrasonic pulse and the pulse repetition frequency. This implies that continuously energized equipment compared to one functioning in a pulsed mode needs to utilize lower amplitude pulses. This is indeed the case as illustrated by the values for the peak pressure given in Table 4 in Chapter 3.

M-mode and pulsed Doppler are two stationary beam examination techniques. The former utilizes short pulses to give good axial resolution and a relatively low pulse repetition frequency. It can therefore use high amplitude pulses, within the bounds set by cavitation consideration limits. Pulsed Doppler uses relatively long pulses to give good spectral resolution and a high pulse repetition frequency to avoid aliasing when measuring fast flow. Modern equipment therefore automatically reduces the amplitude of the pulse when long range-gates and high repetition frequencies are employed.

B-mode and color Doppler imaging are scanned-beam examination techniques. Both utilize short pulses for good axial resolution but, in order to get a stable mean Doppler measurement, the color Doppler technique insonates the same point in tissue by several repetition pulses. Both techniques may employ higher amplitude pulses than stationary beam examination methods, and theoretically B-mode may use pulses with the highest amplitude.

Issues such as these go some way towards explaining the differences in the values of the various acoustic parameters listed in the tables in Chapter 3.

CONCLUSION

The features of an ultrasonic field relevant to its ability to cause a potential bioeffect are currently specified in terms of four acoustic parameters: two related to its ability to heat tissue, and two potentially to cause a cavitationally induced bioeffect. Although the terminology used to describe these parameters is at first sight daunting, once the code used to structure the terminology is appreciated the terms become self-explanatory and descriptive of the features being quantified. All users of ultrasound are encouraged to develop the expertise to appreciate the description of acoustic exposures being generated by their equipment.

References

1. Kremkau, F. W. (1993). *Diagnostic Ultrasound: Principles and Instruments.* (Philadelphia: W. B. Saunders)
2. Naugol'nykh, K. A. and Ostrovsky, L. A. (1994). *Nonlinear Acoustics.* (New York: American Institute of Physics)
3. Preston, R. C. (1991). *Output Measurements for Medical Ultrasound.* (London: Springer-Verlag)
4. Ziskin, M. C. and Lewin, P. A. (1993). *Ultrasonic Exposimetry.* (Boca Raton: CRC Press)
5. Food and Drug Administration (1985). *510(k) Guide for Measuring and Reporting Acoustic Output of Diagnostic Ultrasound,* 1992 updated draft document. Food and Drug Administration, Center for Devices and Radiological Health)

Acoustic output of modern ultrasound equipment: is it increasing?

3

F. A. Duck and J. Henderson

SUMMARY

Standard methods for the measurement of ultrasound exposure have been used for a period of over 20 years to quantify and report the intensities and acoustic pressures used in diagnostic ultrasound. By reviewing the reports of surveys of exposure it is possible to demonstrate a general increasing trend in the average exposure levels over this time, both in time-averaged intensity and in peak acoustic pressure. Of particular note is the high peak intensity introduced by pulsed Doppler operation in the 1980s, with average values of spatial peak temporal average intensity (I_{SPTA}) now over 1 W/cm^2 and with occasional reports of intensities approaching 10 W cm^2. The average intensity depends on the mode of operation. It is lowest for fetal heart monitors, and becomes progressively higher for B-mode imaging, M-mode, Doppler imaging and pulsed Doppler operation, in that order. The average intensity increases for each of the modes listed by a factor of approximately three. There is considerable overlap between the modes with, for example, the highest intensity used for Doppler imaging exceeding the median intensity used for pulsed Doppler operation. There is, however, little difference between the pulse amplitudes used in each of the modes, with the median peak rarefaction pressure a little above 2 MPa for all conditions. The widespread adoption of other means of expressing exposure, the use of estimated *in situ* exposure values and biophysical indices, for example, may cause difficulties in continued monitoring of these trends. The recent relaxation of the regulatory control by the Food and Drug Administration (FDA) in the USA will result in increases in the mean exposures used internationally, especially in obstetrics.

INTRODUCTION

This chapter presents the current knowledge of the acoustic output of contemporary diagnostic ultrasonic equipment. Comparisons are made with exposures from other applications of ultrasound in medicine, therapeutic and surgical uses, for example, in order to place the exposures in some context. Measured and estimated values of acoustic output are given for the variety of imaging modes and transducer types currently available commercially. In addition, the evidence that the exposure of patients to ultrasound has increased over the recent past is evaluated. The reasons for such an increase are reviewed, and ways by which the clinical user may affect the exposure during an ultrasonic examination are explored.

Before presenting tables of values which review the present knowledge of exposure from diagnostic ultrasound, a brief preliminary discussion is necessary to set the scene. (Note that a more detailed description of acoustic parameters that describe ultrasound exposure is given in Chapter 2). The ultrasonic pulse may be described by the use of a number of acoustic quantities, such as power, intensity, acoustic pressure and particle velocity[1], and its structure and size in terms of pulse length, beamwidth and working frequency. It is important to select the acoustic parameters that are most useful in quantifying biological responses to the field, otherwise the ability to make judgements about safety can become unnecessarily complicated. To this end, the amplitude of the pulse itself may be expressed either by the pulse-average intensity (I_{SPPA}) or the peak rarefaction pressure (p_r). Time-averaged quantities that have been chosen are total acoustic power and spatial peak temporal average intensity (I_{SPTA}).

An additional parameter that must be considered when values are used for ultrasonic exposure is whether they are 'free-field' or 'estimated *in situ*'. Free-field exposure measurements are fundamental to all acoustic exposure and represent the acoustic field in water, usually measured by a calibrated hydrophone[2]. The main advantage of these measurements is that they are, in principle, straightforward, and can be readily achieved and repeatedly obtained in independent laboratories. For this reason a substantial independent database of free-field exposure measurements exists in the literature and this may be used to explore changes which may have occurred in ultrasonic output levels, as ultrasound equipment has developed. A major criticism of free-field exposure values is that they give no direct estimation of exposure within the body, except at the surface. Attenuation of the ultrasonic pulse by overlying tissue increases logarithmically with both frequency and depth for a homogeneous tissue. By developing models for exposure circumstances it is possible, in principle, to predict exposure within the body on the basis of the free-field water measurements of exposure. A very simple model[3] has been used by the FDA in the USA as the basis of the regulatory structure which assumes the tissue to be uniform, with an attenuation loss of 0.3 dB/cm per MHz. All exposure values given by manufacturers for ultrasound regulatory purposes include this 'derating' factor.

REVIEW OF MEASUREMENTS OF ACOUSTIC OUTPUT

As commercial systems are developed, enter the market and are replaced, the range of output values alters. Completely up-to-date information summarizing the output is difficult to compile. What follows is drawn together from a few of the most recent publications in which exposure data are summarized either from independent measurements[4–6] or from data provided by manufacturers[7]. Henderson and colleagues[6] evaluated the free-field exposure from 223 probes used with 82 scanning systems in an independent survey of equipment in clinical use in the Northern Regional Health Authority of the British National Health Service. Patton and associates[7] collated data submitted by manufacturers to the FDA in the USA for regulatory purposes. The latter study from a total of about 140 transducers is useful in that it tabulates estimated *in situ* exposures, thermal estimates and thermal index values.

A summary of exposures for diagnostic ultrasound is given in Tables 1–4. For pulsed fields (Tables 1–3) the two quantities relating to pulse

Table 1 Free-field ultrasonic exposure in water from conventional transducers operating in B-mode imaging and M-mode. (All values from reference 6, except I_{SPPA} from reference 5)

Application	Range	Median
Imaging and M-mode		
Peak rarefaction pressure, p_r (MPa)	0.45–5.54	2.4
Spatial peak pulse average intensity, I_{SPPA} (W/cm^2)	14–933	230
M-mode only		
Spatial peak temporal average intensity, I_{SPTA} (mW/cm^2)	11.2–430	106
Acoustic power (mW)	1–68	9
B-mode only		
Spatial peak temporal average intensity, I_{SPTA} (mW/cm^2)	0.3–991	34
Acoustic power (mW)	0.3–285	75

Table 2 Free-field ultrasonic exposure in water from endovaginal probes operating in B-mode imaging and M-mode. (Values from reference 6, except for acoustic power from reference 7 and I_{SPPA} from reference 5)

Application	Range	Median
Imaging and M-mode		
Peak rarefaction pressure, p_r (MPa)	0.66–3.50	2.29
Spatial peak pulse average intensity, I_{SPPA} (W/cm^2)	50–322	244.0
M-mode only		
Spatial peak temporal average intensity, I_{SPTA} (mW/cm^2)	2.0–210	55.7
Acoustic power (mW)	0.35–2.8	0.81
B-mode only		
Spatial peak temporal average intensity, I_{SPTA} (mW/cm^2)	0.8–284	18.8
Acoustic power (mW)	0.61–22	4.6

Table 3 Free-field ultrasonic exposure in water from all transducers operating in pulsed Doppler and color Doppler imaging modes. (Values from reference 6 except I_{SPPA} from reference 5)

	Spectral pulsed Doppler		Color Doppler imaging	
	Range	Median	Range	Median
Peak rarefactional pressure (MPa)	0.67–5.32	2.1	0.46–4.25	2.38
Spatial peak pulse average intensity, I_{SPPA} (W/cm^2)	1.1–771	144.0	60–670	275.0
Spatial peak temporal average intensity, I_{SPTA} (mW/cm^2)	173–9080	1180.0	21–2050	290.0
Acoustic power (mW)	10–440	100.0	15–440	90.0

amplitude are given first, acoustic peak negative pressure (p_r) and pulse average intensity (I_{SPPA}), followed by the two time-averaged quantities acoustic power and temporal-average intensity (I_{SPTA}). B-mode imaging and M-mode exposures are given separately for the time-averaged quantities.

Some general comments about the values may be made. At the outset it should be emphasized that the values summarize the range of highest achievable exposures for any particular transducer and application for all the systems evaluated. Under normal use it may be expected that the machine settings used for each measurement would perhaps be rarely used (the machine factors affecting output are reviewed below). Nevertheless, the values do give valuable information about the acoustic output capable of being generated by present-day diagnostic equipment. There is a wide range of exposure for all transducer types and applications. Peak acoustic pressure varies between about 0.5 and 5.0 MPa, and the intensities typically span two orders of magnitude. Caution is advised when

Table 4 Free-field ultrasonic exposure in water from continuous-wave Doppler systems. (From reference 4). NR, not reported

	Range	Median
Peripheral vascular and cardiac		
Peak pressure (kPa)	18–160	54
Spatial peak temporal average intensity, I_{SPTA} (mW/cm^2)	8.5–850	99
Acoustic power (mW)	2.3–90	16
Fetal heart		
Peak pressure (kPa)	13–31	NR
I_{SPTA} (mW/cm^2)	6–33	NR
Acoustic power (mW)	17–25	NR

the highest values are requoted, since occasionally the most extreme have been revised downwards by manufacturers subsequent to the survey. This does not imply that all equipment in use around the world would have been modified as a result. The fact that these extreme exposures have been observed in surveys stresses the need for vigilance.

Most recent surveys of exposure have quoted both mean and median values; for conciseness here only the median values have been included. Whilst surveys of pulse amplitude parameters, p_r and I_{SPPA}, demonstrate symmetrical distributions of values for which the median and mean values are close, the distributions of time-averaged values, acoustic power and I_{SPTA}, for example, are strongly skewed, with a small number of very high values. For these skewed distributions it is felt that the median, together with a note of the overall range, gives a more representative summary of the exposure. Typical distributions are shown in Figures 1 and 2.

COMPARISON OF MODES OF OPERATION

Values for exposure are given for conventional imaging transducers (Table 1) and for endo-

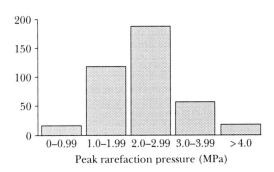

Figure 1 Distribution of free-field peak rarefaction pressure in water from a survey of all pulsed operating modes: B-mode imaging, Doppler imaging and pulsed Doppler. From reference 6

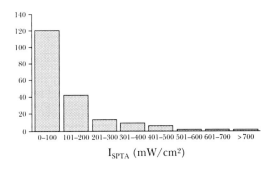

Figure 2 Distribution of free-field spatial peak temporal average intensity (I_{SPTA}) in water from a survey of B-mode imaging. From reference 6

vaginal transducers (Table 2), and Doppler exposures are shown in Tables 3 and 4. Comparison between Tables 1 and 2 shows that the pulse amplitudes being used for vaginal scanning are similar to those used for conventional transducers, although not reaching the very highest values. The time-averaged intensities for vaginal transducers are about 3 dB below those used for conventional scanning, on average[7]. Broadly, this situation is also true when the values are derated at 0.3 dB/cm per MHz. The survey of such derated exposures shows similarly broad equivalence of estimated *in situ* pulse amplitude, with time-averaged exposures up to about 3 dB below those used for conventional imaging. At first sight this may seem surprising in view of the smaller scan depths used for vaginal scanning, but it would appear that this is compensated for by the higher loss from the generally higher frequencies used.

General comparison between modes of operation also demonstrates no difference of any significance between the pulse amplitudes used in any category. In the values tabulated here, the median values vary from 2.1 MPa for pulsed Doppler to 2.4 MPa for imaging within an overall range spanning 0.45–5.54 MPa. This is an important observation, since a view has been held that pulse amplitude is an important exposure parameter only for imaging, and not for other applications. This assertion is not supported by the evidence reported in any survey.

It is for the spatial peak temporal average intensity (I_{SPTA}) that the difference between modes of operation is most marked. In ascending order, the median values of I_{SPTA} are: B-mode (34 mW/cm^2), M-mode (106 mW/cm^2), color Doppler (290 mW/cm^2) and pulsed Doppler (1180 mW/cm^2), each about a factor of 3 above the mode lower. This trend is similarly reflected in the upper and lower values of the ranges of each (see Tables 1 and 3). Whilst acoustic power has been reported, and is included within these tables, there are clear difficulties in its measurement, especially for imaging systems with sector format. Consequently, it is probably a more useful and reliable quantity for the comparison of stationary beams (M-mode and pulsed Doppler) than it is for scanned systems.

A complete review of exposure requires more detail than is given here, and thorough reviews include this detail[4]. For example, the highest reported acoustic pressure measured adjacent to the transducer is 1.51 MPa, with typical values of about 0.5 MPa. Pulse durations for imaging are about 0.5 µs or less, although for pulsed Doppler applications they may reach 15 µs. Pulse repetition frequencies for Doppler can lie anywhere in the range 1–50 kHz. These and other details can be important in evaluation of the relevance of laboratory safety studies to the clinical situation.

Doppler ultrasound output

The potential for pulsed Doppler systems to operate at substantially higher intensities than any other modes was recognized in the mid-1980s when this mode was introduced[8,9], and currently most commercial pulsed Doppler systems can operate at temporally averaged intensities which exceed 1 W/cm^2. The introduction of color Doppler imaging brought with it concerns that this mode, too, would operate at comparably higher intensities. However, the evidence is that, whilst color Doppler indeed operates at intensities about ten times higher than those used for conventional imaging, these are still generally lower than those used in pulsed Doppler. This intermediate position results directly from the method of operation of color Doppler systems, using, as they do, sequences of pulse trains which are scanned throughout the imaged field. Nevertheless, there is a substantial overlap between color Doppler imaging and pulsed Doppler intensities, and at least one color Doppler system was reported as being capable of operating at over 2 W/cm^2.

Monitoring systems

Exposure from continuous wave systems is summarized in Table 4. For clarity, fetal monitoring applications have been separated from other continuous wave Doppler systems, for which considerably higher intensities may be used. Overall, the highest exposures (both power and

I_{SPTA}) occur with Doppler attachments to scanning equipment[4,10]. The pressure amplitudes are about 100 times lower than diagnostic pulse amplitudes, with intensities similar to those used for M-mode. Fetal heart monitors use the lowest pressure amplitudes and peak intensities of all. The highest recorded value of I_{SPTA} in this application is equivalent to the median for imaging, about 30 mW/cm^2.

RELIABILITY OF DATA

Comparison between two recent surveys[6,7] shows that there is still some disagreement in reported values of exposure. The survey carried out by Patton and colleagues[7] draws together values reported to the FDA by manufacturers for regulatory purposes. The procedures used for these measurements are well documented[11], and should have given rise to a set of data of good quality. Similarly, the second survey carried out in the UK by an experienced team, on a wide range of manufactured scanners in clinical use, carries the advantage that standard protocols were used on all scanners, irrespective of their manufacturer[12]. Generally, the water values reported in the USA survey are lower than equivalent values reported in the UK survey, by up to a factor of 2. There could be several contributory causes for this difference, but the most probable explanation relates to the different measurement protocols used in the two surveys. The USA protocol requires that the measurement be carried out at the location where the derated intensity reaches its maximum value. For many reasons this is not where the maximum of any exposure value is reached under the free-field conditions used in the British study. The derating calculation, non-linear propagation effects and beam overlap in imaging all act to alter the relative positions in the field at which any exposure quantity reaches a maximum. If such factors are discounted during the exposure measurement, it is clearly possible for the measurement not to represent the overall free-field maximum achieved in any field. Other factors may also influence the comparison. The selection of equipment was different, although since both studies included over 100 transducers it might be expected that the importance of this would be small. Hydrophones used may have been of inadequate size. If the hydrophone area is comparable with the beam area, spatial averaging gives rise to erroneously low measurements of peak pressure and intensity. Finally, it has recently been noted[13] that it is not uncommon for the conditions giving rise to the overall maximum exposure to be missed by the manufacturers own measurements. Given the extreme complexity of modern systems this is perhaps not surprising, but it nevertheless means that careful independent measurements of exposure can well identify extreme conditions giving rise to higher exposure conditions than those noted and declared by even the most scrupulous of manufacturers.

TRENDS IN EXPOSURE

As the use of ultrasound in diagnostic medicine has developed over the last quarter of a century, reports have appeared in the literature which make it possible to enumerate trends in ultrasonic exposure as equipment and techniques have developed. During the recent past reviews of trends in exposure have been published[4,5] which demonstrate and quantify the progressive increase in average acoustic output of clinical scanners. Hill's first detailed report[14] of diagnostic ultrasound exposures in 1971 used essentially the same measurement devices that are now universally used for exposure measurement: a calibrated hydrophone and a radiation force balance. His study of 15 pulse-echo and three continuous-wave Doppler systems provides a baseline against which subsequent surveys can be judged. The survey of Carson and co-workers[15] about a decade later included both spatially and temporally averaged intensities, so laying the groundwork for the subsequent use of intensities in later work. This survey also included measurements made on early real-time systems. Not long afterwards, the availability of exposure data reported to the FDA in the USA for regulatory purposes enabled Stewart[16] to survey 90 pulse-echo fetal imaging systems. The important observation was the strongly skewed

distribution of intensity, which still exists in current surveys (Figure 2). By the mid-1980s, evidence of a trend towards higher average output was noted in several published reports[9,17]. The American Institute of Ultrasound in Medicine published two reports in 1985 and 1987 giving further manufacturers' data; the first is important in that it is the earliest publication to note the considerably higher intensities used in pulsed Doppler beams[8]. Many of the pulsed Doppler transducers were reported to be operating at I_{SPTA} intensity in excess of 1 W/cm^2, the highest being 1.95 W/cm^2. Since that time there have been a number of reports from many sources reviewing declared or measured output from the full range of diagnostic equipment, from many countries[18]. The latest reports include measurements of exposure from color Doppler systems and from intraluminal transducers.

From these reports, all of which have reported measures of exposure under free-field conditions in water, it is possible to express quantitatively apparent trends in average exposure conditions. The median values for two exposure quantities, peak acoustic pressure and temporal average intensity (I_{SPTA}) have been selected from a set of surveys[5,6,8,9,13–15] to illustrate these trends (Figures 3 and 4). Peak pressure amplitudes used in imaging and M-mode have increased progressively over the two decades under review, resulting in an increase

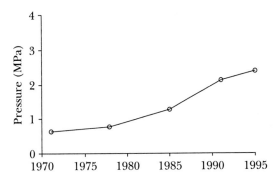

Figure 3 The median values of free-field peak rarefaction pressure for B- and M-modes from surveys covering the period 1970–95, demonstrating a progressive upward trend. References are given in the text

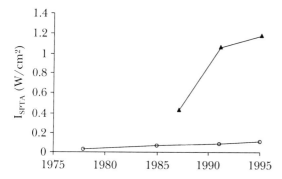

Figure 4 Median values of free-field spatial peak temporal average intensity (I_{SPTA}) for M-mode (circles) and pulsed Doppler (triangles) from surveys covering the period 1975–95. References are given in the text

by a factor of 4 for p_r. As noted above, p_c is less appropriate than p_r to characterize the pulse amplitude, but not surprisingly shows a comparable increase over time[5]. Non-linear propagation effects are important in exposure measurement[19], causing average values of p_c to be about twice those for p_r. Another important outcome of this non-linearity is a phenomenon known as acoustic saturation, important because it sets an absolute upper limit for the pressure amplitude that can be reached for any ultrasonic field[20,21]. Conditions of acoustic saturation are closely approached in water for diagnostic beams currently used at the highest levels, and, as a result, any further increases in source output will be increasingly hidden from hydrophone measurements at the beam focus, because of the increased non-linear loss of energy in the water path[5]. As a result, hydrophone measurements may underestimate the true exposure condition in tissue.

Figure 4 compares trends in peak time-averaged intensities for the two conditions using stationary beams, M-mode and pulsed Doppler. The comparatively low intensities used for M-mode applications have nevertheless shown a progressive trend upwards, the median now being about 100 mW/cm². As noted above, the much higher intensities used in pulsed Doppler beams had already been reported by 1987. Subsequent surveys have shown median intensities slightly above 1 W/cm², an order of magnitude

higher than those used for M-mode applications.

Recently, Henderson and colleagues[6] reported an increase in measured time-averaged intensities in B-mode imaging, giving a range (and median) of 0.3–991 (34.0) mW/cm², about five times greater than intensities reported in a similar survey[5] carried out in 1991. A comparable increase of rather smaller magnitude was noted for color Doppler measurements. No such increases were reported for unscanned beams operating in M-mode and pulsed Doppler mode. The most probable explanation may well lie in the ability of the measurement protocol of Henderson and co-workers to identify more readily the true location of the peak intensity in imaging beams. By integrating the total power in the hydrophone signal[22], it was possible more easily to find the position of greatest intensity, particularly under conditions of considerable beam overlap close to the transducer. It is also important to recognize that the quest for improvements in image quality, and in particular for high spatial resolution in small imaging areas, increases the chance of using higher exposure, because of the greater scan-line density.

Whilst the evidence presented appears strongly to support the assertion of a progressive increase in output, this should not be accepted uncritically. The earlier surveys were of relatively small numbers. It is possible that subsequent surveys, being more extensive, revealed the occasional very high exposure condition which had been missed by earlier smaller surveys. Even so, it is difficult to use this argument to discount the reported trend upwards in *average* exposure values. Improved hydrophone performance and calibration could have had an impact on the quality of measurements. The more resilient international standards for hydrophone calibration give rise to greater confidence in more recent survey results. In addition, the frequency response of modern, polyvinylidene fluoride (pvdf), membrane hydrophones is considerably improved in range and flatness over earlier ceramic probe hydrophones, and this has certainly allowed peak positive pressures to be measured more accurately in non-linearly distorted pulses.

However, for p_r and derived intensities it is unlikely that improved hydrophone bandwidth or calibration has avoided any systematic underestimation of these quantities. One factor that may have improved measurements, particularly in highly focused fields, has been the availability of hydrophones with smaller sensitive areas, measurements from which avoid the spatial averaging which arises from the use of larger hydrophones. For such narrow beams, it may be that earlier measurements underestimated the true peak pressures, and this could be a small contributing factor to the observed trend upwards; later surveys have commonly used hydrophones with standard 0.5-mm diameter active elements.

If the evidence for progressive increases in output is accepted, a brief comment on the mechanisms of control and potential for further increases is pertinent. The regulatory mechanism of any country with a large ultrasound use strongly influences the design of systems. For this reason it has been the regulatory structure of the USA, operating through the FDA, which has been the main steadying hand limiting the output of diagnostic systems. Recent alterations in the process for gaining FDA approval are likely to result in further increases in average exposure values. This has come about from permission to allow higher intensities in some categories including obstetrics, provided safety indices are displayed to the user. Were a decision to be made to relax the FDA structure further still, accepting the display of the thermal index (TI) and mechanical index (MI) as the only necessary safety criterion, then in the absence of internationally accepted alternatives, further increases in output might be expected.

Comparison with other medical ultrasonic exposure

The capability of high ultrasound intensities both to heat and to destroy living tissue allows its use for therapy and for surgery, and it is instructive to compare exposures that are used in these applications with those used in medical diagnosis[4]. Each of the two general categories of exposure, the amplitude of each pulse and the time-averaged intensity, may be compared.

For physiotherapy, ultrasound is generally delivered as a continuous wave, or in long pulses of about a millisecond in duration, about 1000 times longer than those used in diagnostic applications. The beams are unfocused. Current equipment operates with maximum time-averaged intensities, I_{SATA}, of about $3 \, W/cm^2$, and total acoustic power of about 15 W. These exposures are limited under international standards[23,24]. Local peak intensities may be up to 40 times the spatially averaged intensities, because of beam non-uniformity. Under normal clinical use, however, physiotherapy treatments would normally use attenuated machine settings, commonly about $0.5 \, W/cm^2$.

A recent direct comparison has been reported between the ultrasound output from a typical physiotherapy unit and a typical diagnostic scanner operating in pulsed Doppler mode at its highest output[25]. The greatest acoustic power available for pulsed Doppler studies was shown to be equivalent to that used in some physiotherapy applications, and it was noted that the highest peak pressures were reached, not in the physiotherapy fields, but at the focus of the pulsed Doppler beam. It was also noted that physiotherapy equipment is required to operate so that the output automatically stops after a pre-set time period, whereas such a control is not mandatory on diagnostic equipment.

The therapeutic application of ultrasound depends for its effectiveness, at least in part, on local tissue heating and consequent enhancement of perfusion. Continued exposure of tissue to intensities in excess of about $10 \, W/cm^2$ can result in selective destruction of cellular structures, and this has been used in a number of hyperthermic and surgical applications of ultrasound[26], most of which have failed to reach widespread use. At sufficiently high intensities, of the order of $10^3 \, W/cm^2$, lesions may be generated within a few seconds[27].

In extracorporeal lithotripsy the action of ultrasound pulses depends not on the time-averaged intensity but on exposure properties of the pulse itself. In a survey of lithotripsy fields[28], the greatest free-field negative pressures were in the range 3.6–9.9 MPa, overlapping those for diagnostic applications. However, it would be quite false to conclude that the biological effects are therefore equivalent. The pulse energy in lithotripsy is much higher than for any diagnostic application, reaching a maximum of 90 mJ per pulse, and the center frequency of a lithotripsy pulse is about 10 times lower than that for imaging.

CONTROL OF EXPOSURE BY THE OPERATOR

It has been frequently noted that the exposures documented in surveys are the greatest values determined by measurement, by exploring all the alternative settings on a machine. Conversely, of course, the operator may be unlikely to use the particular condition identified as generating the greatest pressure or intensity. One purpose of the so-called output display standard[29] is to give information to the operator about the way in which the particular settings of the scanner affect the output during scanning. To assist in understanding, it is worth reviewing in outline here the most important ways in which exposure is altered by scanner controls. A similar review is given elsewhere[30].

For any transducer, the three factors that dominate any considerations of operational exposure are the scan mode, the output control and the dwell time. As this chapter has shown, the pulse amplitude is not primarily affected by the mode selected, whereas the time-averaged intensity depends strongly upon it. Most notably, the selection of pulsed Doppler mode will invariably dominate time-averaged intensity. If several modes are being operated simultaneously, the intensity will depend on technical details of pulse interleaving; to a first approximation the intensity of the highest mode may be assumed.

The output control affects both pulse amplitude and intensity. For many systems imaging and Doppler outputs are controlled separately, and users need to be aware of the characteristics of their own machine controls. Output for each can, in principle, be set below maximum by an appropriate start-up protocol, and increased from this only when required. Only the simplest modern scanners have no imaging output control, although some complex scanners lack a Doppler output control. It is important to distinguish on each machine between the output control and the receiver gain control, since both affect the image in a similar way, and sometimes the labelling is misleading. Dwell time is entirely under operator control, and is not considered in any exposure measurement protocol, for which the transducer is assumed not to move, giving an infinite dwell time. Its relative importance derives from considerations of the looked-for effect: cavitation can occur within a pulse period, and so dwell time is of small importance; streaming rise-times are of the order of a second, and thermal rise-times of the order of a minute, and beams moved within these times will result in smaller biophysical effects.

Other front-panel controls may also affect the output in rather more subtle ways, which often depend upon the particular design of the scanner itself. For example, in pulsed Doppler mode, the acoustic pulse-train commonly changes as the sample volume and blood velocity range values are altered. Acoustic pulse length may change with sample volume, and pulse repetition frequency depends on velocity range. Limits are applied to total acoustic power on commercial equipment to ensure that pulse repetition frequency and pulse length alterations do not result in excessive output, and this is done by lowering pulse amplitude when either pulse repetition frequency or pulse length are increased. As a result the highest pulse amplitudes on Doppler applications are often used when a combined small sample volume and low velocity range are used. Similar considerations may apply in color Doppler applications.

For some systems the total acoustic power alters depending on the selection of the focal depth, resulting in the greatest powers being used with the deepest foci. This can be true for both imaging and Doppler systems. Further examples of more subtle effects occur in imaging, when the time-averaged intensity may be increased by both frame rate and scan line density. This may happen when using high-resolution, magnification or zoom modes, when a field of view of limited width is selected.

In summary, documented exposure information given to users can provide only an overview of the worst-case conditions pertaining to a particular transducer and scanner. The user should be aware that it is possible to use lower exposures than these, and that several of the front-panel controls on the scanner alter the exposures being used. On-line displays of output quantities can be helpful in guiding the user's understanding of the way in which output is altered by the machine settings being selected during scanning.

References

1. Duck, F. A. (1987). The measurement of exposure to ultrasound and its application to estimates of ultrasound 'dose'. *Phys. Med. Biol.*, **32**, 303–25
2. International Electrotechnical Commission (1992). *IEC 1157, Requirements for the declaration of the acoustic output of medical diagnostic ultrasonic equipment.* (Geneva: International Electrotechnical Commission)
3. US Department of Health and Human Services, Food and Drug Administration (1993). *Revised 510(k) Diagnostic Ultrasound Guidance for 1993.* (Rockville, MD: Food and Drug Administration)
4. Duck, F. A. and Martin., K. (1992). Exposure values for medical devices. In Ziskin, M. and Lewin, P. (eds.) *Ultrasonic Exposimetry*, pp. 315–44. (Boca Raton: CRC Press)
5. Duck, F. A. and Martin, K. (1991). Trends in diagnostic ultrasound exposure. *Phys. Med. Biol.*, **36**, 1423–32
6. Henderson, J., Willson, K., Jago, J. R. and Whittingham, T. A. (1995). A survey of the acoustic outputs of diagnostic ultrasound equipment in current clinical use in the Northern Region. *Ultrasound Med. Biol.*, **21**, 699–705
7. Patton, C. A., Harris, G. R. and Phillips, R. A. (1994). Output levels and bioeffects indices from diagnostic ultrasound exposure data reported to the FDA. *IEEE Trans. Ultrasonics Ferroelectrics and Freq. Contr.*, **41**, 353–9
8. American Institute of Ultrasound in Medicine (1985). *Acoustical Data for Diagnostic Equipment.* (Rockville, Maryland: AIUM)
9. Duck, F. A., Starritt, H. C., Aindow, J. D., Perkins, M. A. and Hawkins, A. J. (1985). The output of pulse-echo ultrasound equipment: a survey of powers, pressures and intensities. *Br. J. Radiol.*, **58**, 989–1001
10. Duck, F. A., Starritt, H. C. and Anderson, S. P. (1987). A survey of the acoustic output of ultrasonic Doppler equipment. *Clin. Phys. Physiol. Meas.*, **8**, 39–49
11. National Electrical Manufacturers Association (1992). *Acoustic Output Measurement Standards Publication No. UD-2.* (Washington, DC: NEMA)
12. Henderson, J., Jago, J. R., Willson, K. and Whittingham, T. A. (1993). Towards a protocol for measurement of maximum spatial peak temporal average intensity from diagnostic B mode scanners in the field. *Phys. Med. Biol.*, **38**, 1611–22
13. Jago, J. R., Henderson, J., Whittingham, T. A. and Willson, K. (1995). How reliable are manufacturer's reported acoustic output data? *Ultrasound Med. Biol.*, **21**, 135–6
14. Hill, C. R. (1971). Acoustic intensity measurements on ultrasonic devices. In Bock, J. and Ossonig, J. (eds.) *Ultrasonographica Medica, Proceedings of the 1st Congress on Medical Ultrasonics*, vol. 2, pp. 21–7. (Vienna: Vienna Academy of Medicine)
15. Carson, P. L., Fischella, P. R. and Oughton, T. V. (1978). Ultrasonic power and intensities produced by ultrasonic diagnostic ultrasound equipment. *Ultrasound Med. Biol.*, **3**, 341–50
16. Stewart, H. F. (1982). Ultrasonic measurement techniques and equipment output levels. In Benwell, D.A. and Repacholi, M. (eds.) *Essentials of Medical Ultrasound*, pp. 77–116. (Clifton, New Jersey: Humana Press)
17. Stewart, H. F. (1983). Output levels from commercial diagnostic ultrasound equipment. *J. Ultrasound Med.*, **2**, 39
18. World Federation of Ultrasound in Medicine and Biology (1989). In Kossoff, G. and Nyborg, W. L. (eds.) Symposium on Safety and Standardisation in Medical Ultrasound. *Ultrasound Med. Biol.*, **15** (Suppl. 1), 47–65
19. Duck, F. A. and Starritt, H. C. (1984). Acoustic shock generation by ultrasonic imaging equipment. *Br. J. Radiol.*, **57**, 231–40
20. Duck, F. A. and Perkins, M. A. (1988). Amplitude-dependent losses in ultrasound exposure measurement. *IEEE Trans. Ultrasonics Ferroelec. Freq. Control*, **UFFC-35**, 232–41

21. Starritt, H. C. and Duck, F. A. (1992). Quantification of acoustic shock in routine exposure measurement. *Ultrasound Med. Biol.*, **18**, 513–15

22. Martin, K. (1988). Measurement of acoustic power parameters from medical ultrasound devices with an RF power meter system. *IEEE Trans. Ultrasonics Ferroelec. Freq. Control*, **UFFC-35**, 140–5

23. International Electrotechnical Commission (1984). *IEC 601-2-5 Medical Electrical Equipment*, Part 2, Particular requirements for safety, Section 2.5, Specification for the safety of ultrasonic therapy equipment. (Geneva: IEC)

24. International Electrotechnical Commission (1996). *International Standard Committee Draft, IEC 1689, Ultrasonics – Physiotherapy systems – Performance requirements and methods of measurement in the frequency range 0.5 MHz to 5 MHz.* (Geneva: IEC)

25. Starritt, H. C. and Duck, F. A. (1992). A comparison of ultrasound exposure in therapy and pulsed Doppler fields. *Br. J. Radiol.*, **65**, 557–63

26. Nussbaum, G. H. (ed.) (1982). *Physical Aspects of Hyperthermia*, Medical Physics Monograph No.8. (New York: American Institute of Physics)

27. Vykhodtseva, N. I., Hynynen, K. and Damianou, C. (1994). Pulse duration and peak intensity during focused ultrasound surgery: theoretical and experimental effects in rabbit brain *in vivo*. *Ultrasound Med. Biol.*, **20**, 987–1000

28. Coleman, A. J. and Saunders, J. E. (1989). A survey of the acoustic output of commercial extracorporeal shock wave lithotripters. *Ultrasound Med. Biol.*, **15**, 213–27

29. American Institute of Ultrasound in Medicine/National Electrical Manufacturers Association (1992). *Standard for Real-Time Display of Thermal and Mechanical Acoustic Output Indices on Diagnostic Ultrasound Equipment.* (Rockville, Maryland: AIUM)

30. Docker, M. F. and Duck, F. A. (eds.) (1991). *The Safe Use of Diagnostic Ultrasound.* (London: British Institute of Radiology)

Can diagnostic ultrasound heat tissue and cause biological effects?

4

S. B. Barnett

SUMMARY

The question raised in this chapter is: 'can diagnostic ultrasound heat tissue and cause biological effects'? The simple answer is, 'yes'. However, this needs to be qualified, as not all ultrasonographic examinations involve a risk of heating. Simple B-mode imaging applies relatively low acoustic outputs and operates with the ultrasound beam briefly scanning through tissues of interest. Such exposures are not capable of producing harmful temperature increases. Evidence from animal studies shows that when diagnostic ultrasound is used in pulsed Doppler mode, fetal tissue near bone can be heated to levels that are biologically significant. It is important in these applications to minimize the acoustic output and duration of exposure.

Thresholds for teratogenic effects of hyperthermia are determined by a combination of the induced temperature elevation and its duration. Most ultrasound diagnostic procedures involve brief dwell times, which help to widen the safety margin. A diagnostic exposure that produces a maximum temperature rise of 1.5 °C above normal physiological levels (37 °C) does not present a risk from thermal effects in humans, regardless of the duration of exposure.

Results of a number of studies on rats and mice have demonstrated that exposure for 5 min to an increase of 4 °C above their normal body temperature is hazardous to embryonic and fetal development. There are few data on the biological effects of interaction of ultrasound with tissues that have a pre-existing temperature elevation. The results of specialized studies using rat embryo culture techniques imply that ultrasound-induced biological effects can be potentiated by an existing elevated core temperature; however, uncertainties remain about the possibility of synergistic effects from such ultrasound interactions.

There are uncertainties in predicting an *in situ* temperature increase in the embryo and fetus. It is therefore, prudent to use the minimum output consistent with obtaining the required diagnostic information and to minimize the duration of pulsed Doppler examinations in pregnancy.

INTRODUCTION

During clinical ultrasonographic examinations acoustic energy is transmitted into the body and interacts with its tissues in ways that may result in a measurable biological response. Currently, the best understood mechanism of interaction is that involving heating. Some of the ultrasound energy is reflected back from interfaces between biological tissues to produce the echographic images, while some of the energy is absorbed and converted to heat. The amount of heat generated is mostly dependent upon the ability of the tissue to absorb, rather than reflect or disperse, ultrasonic energy (i.e. its absorption coefficient) and this is a function of its gross molecular structure. Generally, more dense materials such as bone and teeth have high acoustic absorption coefficients and are, therefore, heated to a greater extent than soft tissue. The absorption coefficient of bone is at least 30 times greater than that of most soft tissue. Amongst soft tissue, proteins with large molecules, such as collagen, also have a relatively high absorption coefficient. An important factor for the induction of biological effects is the rate of ultrasound-induced heating. The speed of heat deposition in bone can be as much as 50 times faster than in soft tissue. Therefore, from a safety perspective, the tissue that has the greatest potential for bioeffects from ultrasound-induced heating is bone, or developing bone. Tissues lying close to, or in contact with bone are also at risk of significant heating by conduction from the bone. Actively dividing tissue is most susceptible to damage by heat. Therefore, situations in which cell division and growth occur close to bone represent a potential risk. Depending on the severity of the effect or the sensitivity of the tissue, this may create a risk to the patient. The extent of risk depends on both the acoustic and the biological properties, i.e. the acoustic exposure conditions and the sensitivity of the target.

When ultrasound energy is absorbed it is transformed into heat and can travel to adjacent tissues, outside the beam, by conduction. The width of the ultrasound beam determines the size of the heated volume, and the amount of heating achieved is limited by dissipating effects of conduction or vascular perfusion. Narrow focussed beams that are typically used in diagnostic applications have a large temperature gradient between the center of the beam and the surrounding tissue, so that heat is rapidly dissipated by conduction[1]. The extent of vascular development largely determines the cooling efficiency, so that highly vascular organs such as the liver or kidney would be less susceptible to heating than bone, which has relatively poorly developed vascularization.

The acoustic outputs of ultrasound scanners in clinical use have increased substantially in recent years (see Chapter 3) and are now capable of producing significant heating effects in some applications. While the risk of thermally related bioeffects is increasing there are changes proposed that may impact on the international regulation of exposure from diagnostic equipment and will place greater responsibility on the user for exposure control and risk assessment. The trend for increasing acoustic output was publicized in a report showing that since 1991 the measured spatial peak temporal average intensity (I_{SPTA}) from diagnostic equipment

in current clinical use in the UK had increased by a factor of approximately five in B-mode applications[2] (refer to Chapter 3 for more detailed information on the current levels of exposure from diagnostic equipment). The total acoustic power output has doubled in pulsed Doppler mode during that period. The importance of this is that the trend for increased acoustic output has now achieved levels where bioeffects can be produced. Ultrasound safety committees and authorities now need to be quite careful in commenting on safety issues and to qualify statements by referring to the clinical significance of observed effects.

ESTIMATED ULTRASOUND-INDUCED TEMPERATURE INCREASE

A large amount of data has been published on the estimated temperature elevation in tissue resulting from exposure by diagnostic ultrasound equipment. One theoretical model[1] developed by the National Council for Radiation Protection and Measurement (NCRP) estimated the worst-case steady state heating that would never be exceeded in diagnostic ultrasound examinations. Another model proposed by the American Institute of Ultrasound in Medicine and the National Electrical Manufacturers Association (AIUM/NEMA)[3] estimated values that are not expected to be exceeded in the majority of ultrasonographic examinations and which were derived using a tissue path attenuation coefficient of 0.3 dB/cm per MHz. The AIUM/NEMA model provides estimates known as the thermal index (TI) that may be displayed during equipment operation. This provides the operator with a relative value from which assumptions may be made about the risk of producing a thermally related bioeffect during an ultrasonographic examination (this USA regulatory aspect is described in more detail in Chapter 12). The estimation of in situ temperature is an extremely complex problem and relies on assumptions about the tissue properties. The presence of such uncertainties gives favor to the concept of a relative index rather than the expectation of an absolute value of the temperature *in situ*.

Soft tissue model

In the first-trimester obstetric scanning by the transabdominal approach, the ultrasound beam passes through layers of maternal tissue before encountering the embryo or early fetus. Hence, a soft (homogeneous) tissue model has been developed[1]. In this situation, the energy in the ultrasound beam is attenuated as it passes through the tissue overlying the obstetric target. At the same time, the intensity increases as the beam focus is approached. As a result, there may be two peaks in the maximum temperature increase; one close to the transducer and a second peak near the focus. The contribution to the maximum temperature increase in soft tissue from self-heating of the transducer is an important factor that the thermal index does not specifically address.

When the liquid-filled maternal bladder is used to provide an 'acoustic window' of low attenuation pathway to the embryo or fetus, the target tissue is heated to a greater extent.

First trimester

The NCRP model was used to estimate the worst-case temperature increases in obstetric examinations based on the maximum outputs of pulsed Doppler (non-fetal) equipment used in Canada[4]. The largest calculated value for the first trimester of pregnancy was 1.6 °C, but the majority of exposures gave a maximum increase in temperature (ΔT_{lim}) of less than 1 °C. A more recent consensus of the AIUM Bioeffects Committee[5] was that for equipment operating at the Food and Drug Administration (FDA)-regulated intensity limit of $I_{SPTA} = 720 \text{ mW/cm}^2$ (derated) the maximum temperature rise in the conceptus could exceed 2 °C.

Fetus

When bone is intercepted by the ultrasound beam the ultrasound-induced temperature rise is substantially increased. It is during obstetric scanning in the second and third trimester when the acoustic beam travels through maternal soft tissue or urine for a fixed distance before impinging on fetal bone. Bly and colleagues[4] calculated ΔT_{lim} of 8.7 °C in the third trimester using the worst-case fixed path attenuation model. Patton and associates[6] calculated the worst-case temperature increase in bone (ΔT_{Blim}) for fetal exposures to be 5.9 °C. This was based on output data obtained from diagnostic equipment approved by the FDA under section 510(k) requirements during the period 1990 to 1991.

MEASURED ULTRASOUND-INDUCED TEMPERATURE INCREASE

In vitro studies

A number of studies have been carried out to quantify ultrasound-induced temperature increase in tissue under simplified, stable experimental conditions where there is no blood flow. These studies use (1) specimens of dead soft tissue exposed in test tanks; (2) specimens of bone exposed in test tanks; and (3) models of gel materials and bone that mimic biological tissue.

Soft tissue

Exposures from commercial equipment or laboratory instruments simulating diagnostic scanners have produced substantial temperature increases in biological tissues when used in pulsed Doppler mode. Consistent results have been reported in unperfused tissues. Exposure conditions of a 5-MHz mechanical sector scanner (beamwidth = 1.9 mm, $I_{SPTA} = 2.0 \text{ W/cm}^2$) gave a maximum temperature increase of 1.9 °C after 2 min in fresh pig liver[7]. With the use of similar equipment, the maximum temperature increase in freshly excised sheep brain was found to be 2.5 °C after 5 min exposure[8]. Exposure in a water tank to 3.2 MHz (simulated pulsed Doppler, -6 dB beamwidth = 2.5 mm, $I_{SPTA} = 2.95 \text{ W/cm}^2$) increased the temperature in freshly excised guinea-pig brain by 2.5 °C after 2 min[9]. These experiments in excised tissue do not allow for cooling by vascular perfusion.

Bone

Greater temperature increases occur when bone is situated within the ultrasound beam. Temperature increases of approximately 5 °C have been reported at the brain/bone tissue interface close to the inner aspect of the skull parietal bone in guinea-pig fetuses[9]. Similar results (temperature increase of 5.1 °C) were recorded using the same exposure conditions in dead guinea-pig fetuses[10]. The amount of ultrasound-induced temperature elevation depended on the fetal gestational age[9]; bone becomes denser and thicker with advancing fetal development. This effect was also demonstrated in insonated specimens of human fetal femurs[11].

Tissue-mimicking phantoms

Water-based gels have been used in experimental systems to provide a homogeneous material with acoustic properties similar to soft tissue. For heating due to ultrasound absorption at or near to the geometric focus, Wu and co-workers[12] reported reasonable agreement between measured and predicted values using the NCRP model, within the range of 1–3.5 MHz. A similar result was reported[13] when measurements at a bone sample in soft tissue-mimicking medium were compared to the worst-case estimated value for unscanned beams.

A study reported measured temperature rise in a piece of human temporal bone embedded in gel[14] exposed to the output from a HP Sonos 1000 diagnostic imaging system. The equipment was operated at a frequency of 2 MHz in combined (color, sector, pulsed Doppler) modes and gave a measured total power output of up to 295 mW. With the transducer positioned 0.2 cm from the phantom a maximum steady-state temperature increase of 11 °C above ambient (20 °C) was measured on the external surface of the temporal bone. An increase of 8 °C was recorded on the internal aspect. The heat generated in bone was reduced by 33% when the water path distance between the transducer and phantom was increased by 1 cm, i.e. closer to an *in utero* exposure condition. It should be

noted that this study[14] used human temporal bone that had been embalmed for 2 years. This process causes leaching of mineral content from the bone and may also alter the geometric patterns of the trabecular bone so that the results obtained might considerably underestimate those occurring with fresh vital human skull bone.

In vivo studies

Fetal head

The susceptibility of the central nervous system (CNS) to damage by increased temperature creates particular interest in measurements of heating at the bone interface and in adjacent brain tissue. With the mouse skull used as a model for human fetal insonations[15] temperature elevations greater than 5 °C were recorded after 90 s in anesthetized animals exposed to either continuous wave or pulsed wave ultrasound at an intensity (I_{SPTA}) of 1.5 W/cm^2. The largest temperature increase was observed in older mice and approached 4 °C within 15 s. The −6 dB focal beamwidth was 2.75 mm. Ultrasound-induced temperature increase measured after death was approximately 10% higher, indicating that blood perfusion in the living animal provided a modest cooling effect to counteract the heating. Similar results were reported showing little difference in ΔT measured at the skull/brain interface before and after death in guinea-pig fetuses insonated *in utero* at 57–61 dga (day of gestational age)[16]. A mean temperature increase of 4.9 °C was measured at the inner aspect of the skull parietal bone of 60 dga fetuses during exposure to 2.5 W/cm^2 of I_{SPTA} for 120 s. In older fetuses near to term (62–67 days of gestation) the mean temperature increase was reduced by approximately 12% to 4.3 °C as a result of cooling from more substantially developed cerebral vasculature (Figure 1). The −6 dB beamwidth was 2.7 mm. The acoustic exposure conditions were within the range of outputs of modern ultrasonographic equipment.

In experiments using a relatively large beam (−6 dB beamwidth of 16 mm), the cooling effects of vascular perfusion were found to limit

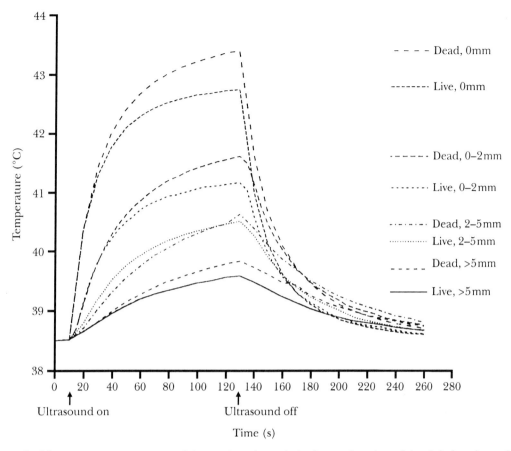

Figure 1 Mean temperature measured *in utero* in guinea-pig brain as a function of depth below the parietal bone. Fetal guinea pigs in the age range 62–66 days of gestation were insonated with 240 mW ultrasound focused on the skull. (From reference 18)

the magnitude of temperature increase in the cerebral cortex in sheep fetuses insonated *in utero*[17]. Exposure to 0.3 W/cm^2 spatial average, temporal average intensity (I_{SATA}) for 120 s produced a mean temperature increase of 1.7 °C which was approximately 40% lower than the post-mortem, non-perfused value. In this study thermocouples and a transducer were surgically attached to the fetal skull and insonation was applied after a recovery period of approximately 7 days. Hence, ultrasound was applied during the normal behavioral state without the need for anesthesia. Temperature was measured in soft tissue at a depth of 1–2 mm from the parietal skull bone.

It is important to know the extent of temperature increase that can be produced in the brain tissue in the first few millimeters of depth in the cerebral cortex, where neural tissue growth continues during fetal development. Horder and co-workers[18] measured the temperature in guinea-pig fetuses in the uterus during insonation and found a mean temperature increase of 2 °C after 120 s at depths of 2–5 mm in the brain. Another study measured temperature in the intracranial cavity in fetuses of second- and third-trimester (ketamine-sedated) monkeys during insonation from a diagnostic scanner[19]. The measurement protocol differed in a number of ways from other studies: temperature was measured by inserting and removing a thermocouple during ultrasound exposure; both the thermocouple and the transducer were manually held in place by the operator during the procedure. This would make precise location of the center of the ultrasound beam extremely difficult. A thermocouple was inserted to a depth of 3.6–4.6 cm in the left cerebral hemisphere of the brain. The greatest temperature elevation recorded was 0.6 °C and this did not differ between pulsed Doppler and B-mode imaging. It should be noted that the quoted I_{SPTA} (in water) values were 54 and 27 mW/cm^2, respectively. These output values are low compared to the maximum free field values recently reported[2] for current equipment; pulsed Doppler $\approx$ 9000 mW/cm^2 and B-mode $\approx$ 990 mW/cm^2. (Refer to Chapter 3 for more information on acoustic outputs of modern equipment.)

BIOLOGICAL EFFECTS OF HYPERTHERMIA

From the scientific data on biological effects of hyperthermia it is generally accepted that tissues containing a large component of actively dividing cells are sensitive to the effects of heat. Abnormalities in cellular physiology and biochemical processes can occur following exposure to increased temperatures above normal basal levels. The interference with normal rates of enzyme synthesis and reactions can affect the way cells grow and divide and may even lead to abnormalities in DNA synthesis and repair processes. Commonly reported effects of heating on embryonic development are the apparent retardation of growth of systems such as the heart, brain[8] and skeleton[20]. Non-specific effects reported as generalized fetal weight reduction are also associated with intrauterine heating or maternal stress.

Developing embryos may mount a protective response to adverse sublethal environmental conditions, such as hyperthermia, that temporarily arrest the process of normal cell division, or mitosis. This phenomenon has been observed in the brains of rodents where normal cell division lapsed for up to 8 h following a single heat treatment[21,22]. Meanwhile, heat shock proteins may be synthesized at the expense of normal neural proteins. On recovery, normal cell division resumed with the fetus appearing morphologically normal, albeit smaller and with a substantial neural deficit.

In embryonic development a lapse of a few hours can lead to substantial delay or disturbance in neurological development. Non-deforming retardation of brain growth and reduced learning performance are common abnormalities in the offspring of moderately heat exposed pregnant guinea pigs. These defects can be caused both during early and during later fetal growth[23]. In general, embryos are more susceptible to damage than fetuses, owing to the high rate of cellular activity during organogenesis. However, continually developing organ systems such as the brain remain susceptible to heat throughout pregnancy. Gross malformations commonly reported include anencephaly, microphthalmia, micrencephaly, maxillary hypoplasia and facial clefting[23]. These results are statistically robust and repeatable, and the bioeffects are irreparable.

Thresholds for biological effects

The effects of increased temperature on biological systems have been extensively reviewed[1,8,23–25]. Whilst many studies have demonstrated that hyperthermia is a common teratogen, the important question to be answered relates to the duration and degree of exposure required to produce the effect.

Animal studies reporting effects of whole-body temperature elevations of approximately 2 °C typically involved exposure to hot air for periods of 60 min because it takes about 30 min to overcome the normal maternal homeostatic response and elevate the maternal core temperature. Studies with rats have reported time constants of the order of 13 min per 1 °C elevation in core temperature[20]. This is a slow rate of heating compared to that caused by ultrasound absorption where substantial elevations occur within seconds. Most early whole-body heating studies were not designed *a priori* to identify threshold levels but, instead, set out to demonstrate that severe developmental abnormalities can be produced by heat exposure. In most cases neither the temperature elevation nor the duration of hyperthermic exposure within the fetus was measured. The heat dose was estimated from the maternal core temperature measured *per rectum*.

A study that was designed to identify a threshold of heat exposure used water immersion body heating and the development of encephaloceles in rats as a gross endpoint[26]. The resting temperature for rats was established from measurement of the core temperature of 50 rats during daylight (i.e. when less active, resting) and gave a mean value of 38.5 ± 0.5 °C. The results of heating found the shortest exposure to be 1 min at a temperature of 43.5 °C (i.e. a 5 °C increase above the normal resting temperature for pregnant rats). The same brain abnormality was observed after 5 min exposure to a temperature elevation of 4 °C.

This threshold for abnormal development in rats (core temperature elevation of 4 °C maintained for 5 min) was subsequently confirmed[27] in a study where hyperthermia was achieved using a water bath. The majority of malformations involved microphthalmia and encephaloceles. The resting core temperature measured in all rats prior to heat treatment was between 38 and 39 °C.

Other studies have also reported development of a major brain abnormality, exencephaly, in mice[28] following intrauterine exposure for 5 min at 42.3 °C. This is an increase of 4.3 °C above the normal body temperature of mice. This was subsequently confirmed when Shiota[29] reported a threshold for exencephaly in mice as being 5 min at a temperature increase of 4.5 °C above their normal body temperature. An exposure to a temperature increase of 3.5 °C above normal for 10 min produced exencephaly in mice[29] and microphthalmia in rats[30] following whole-body hyperthermia.

The rapid onset of ultrasound-induced heating and its related bioeffects was demonstrated in a study showing abnormalities in proliferating bone marrow cells in adult guinea pigs following exposure to localized hyperthermia. An original study heated animals to 42.5–43.5 °C in a hot air incubator for 60 min and reported abnormal nuclear division and growth in neutrophils[31]. When ultrasound was used to elevate the temperature in the marrow, the same cellular abnormalities were observed following exposures to 43 °C (i.e. a temperature increase of 3.5 °C above normal body temperature for guinea pigs) for 4 min[32]. Figure 2 shows the typical bizarre multi-segmented nuclei in neutrophils obtained in a smear of bone marrow taken 2 h after the ultrasound exposure.

There is evidence from sensitive studies using embryo culture systems that the effects of ultrasound may be enhanced by a moderate temperature increase[33,34]. The exposure conditions were a temperature increase of 1.5 °C (absolute temperature 40 °C) together with an ultrasound I_{SPTA} intensity of 1.2 W/cm^2 applied for 15 min duration.

Evidence from repeated studies in different animal species shows that major maldevelopment of brain structure occurs after exposure to a temperature increase of 4 °C for 5 min. The same exposure threshold was found for ultrasound-induced temperature increase on proliferating bone marrow cells[32].

CLINICAL SIGNIFICANCE

Exposure to some diagnostic equipment operating in pulsed Doppler mode has been shown to produce biologically-significant temperature increases in tissue, particularly when bone is present. The biological consequences of a hyperthermic episode depend on the magnitude of temperature elevation and the duration of exposure. Data are available for whole-body exposures (generally resulting in severe abnormalities) where it has been shown that rat embryos exposed to a temperature increase of 4 °C for 5 min developed encephaloceles[23,26].

Under the current FDA (Food and Drug Administration regulator of Radiation Devices and Health) Track 3 option, manufacturers in the USA may obtain market approval for equipment with an output display where the only limit is a maximum I_{SPTA} intensity (derated at the point of interest in tissue) of 720 mW/cm^2. This means that fetal exposures can be increased by almost a factor of 8 above that approved under the alternative application-specific intensity limits that apply in the USA. This could occur with multi-mode imaging systems. Note that the

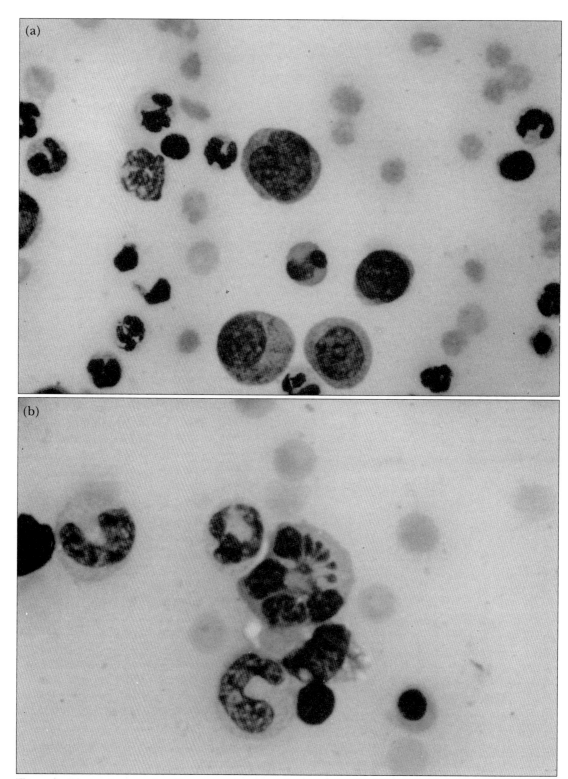

Figure 2 Photomicrograph of bone marrow smear from guinea-pig femur, showing characteristic multisegmented nuclei in neutrophils 2 h after exposure to ultrasound-induced temperature increase. a, normal cells from control femur; b, ultrasound-exposed cells

fetal body temperature is reported to be normally about 0.5 °C higher than the maternal temperature in humans[35,36].

Hyperthermia is a proven teratogen in mammalian biological systems[23,37,38]. Many of the abnormalities reported in heat-exposed animals have also been found in children following *in utero* febrile episodes[39]. Therefore, heat exposure is considered to be a human teratogen[30,40,41]. Smith and co-workers[42] reported that maternal febrile illness that caused the human body temperature to rise above 38.9 °C in early stages of pregnancy was associated with fetal anomalies. Long-term hyperthermia above 39 °C may therefore be teratogenic to the human fetus. Data from retrospective studies indicate that mothers of babies with various CNS malformations experienced increased prevalence of febrile illness during early pregnancy[43–46].

There are many reports of gross effects of hyperthermia on prenatal development in animals. Hyperthermia is recognized as a potential human teratogen and it is probable that the same effects would occur following exposure to similar elevations of temperature above normal physiological levels. The scale of the effect may be expected to be less in human exposures, owing to the ratio of embryonic/fetal body size to beamwidth. However, subcellular effects of heating within the intense focal zone of ultrasound beams have not been adequately studied. The effect of hyperthermia is dependent on a combination of temperature rise and the duration for which it is maintained. The lowest exposure conditions producing repeatedly observed major malformations in embryonic development is 4 °C for 5 min, applied at a specific sensitive stage in embryonic development prior to organogenesis.

The transducer is a substantial source of heating, by conduction, in soft tissue examinations[8,12]. This is particularly important for pulsed transducers which are inefficient in converting electrical to acoustic energy. Heating is localized close to the transducer. This has implications for safety for intracavitary applications, particularly where there is a trend towards increased power outputs in gynecological examinations using the endovaginal route. The risk of inadvertently exposing an unknown pregnancy to heat cannot be excluded.

International committees and working groups are currently developing test objects to measure the maximum temperature elevations in fields emitted by diagnostic scanners in ways that model clinical applications. Estimates of risk based on whole-body heating do not give any information on the probable potentiating effects of ultrasound interactions when accompanied by moderate temperature elevations.

Estimates of risk are mostly based on existing data on whole-body heat exposure in animal studies. The effects on cell development may be different for the rapid onset of ultrasound-induced heating. Acoustic absorption is immediate, resulting in deep tissue temperature elevation within seconds of exposure, compared to tens of minutes required to elevate fetal temperature under whole-body heating conditions. Therefore, any potential protective mechanism mounted by cell reactions to whole-body hyperthermia would be overridden in ultrasound-induced heating. The degree of temperature elevation is directly dependent on the acoustic absorption coefficient of the target tissue. A further complication is the extent of heating. The heated tissue volume is small and usually restricted to a volume of less than 0.5 cm^3; it is limited by the size of the ultrasound beam. In scanned beams used in imaging procedures any single tissue target is interrogated for only fractions of a second each time the beam sweeps past. Therefore, there is little opportunity to heat a specific tissue target. To achieve significant amounts of heating requires that the ultrasound beam be fixed in relation to a tissue target so that all the energy in the beam is directed onto that target. This occurs in pulsed Doppler spectral measurement techniques.

The effects of damaging a small volume depend on the sensitivity of the target tissue. It is questionable whether or not the effects of damage to small discrete areas of neural tissue would ever be detected by studies of gross morphological structure (see Chapter 6 for more information on the sensitivity of biological tissue to ultrasound). Techniques in molecular biology are more sensitive and need to be adapted to provide assays to detect such small biological effects.

The World Federation for Ultrasound in Medicine and Biology (WFUMB) has sponsored a series of symposia on the safety of ultrasound in medicine. These symposia have involved in-depth discussion and evaluation of the scientific data leading to the formulation of international consensus on the bioeffects and safety of diag-nostic ultrasound[1]. A selection of relevant pub-lished recommendations on the safety of diag-nostic applications with regard to heating effects of ultrasound is given below.

International Guidelines on Safety with regard to Thermal Issues: WFUMB Recommendations (1992)

B-mode imaging

Known diagnostic ultrasound equipment as used today for simple B-mode imaging operates at acoustic outputs that are not capable of pro-ducing harmful temperature rises. Its use in medicine is therefore not contraindicated on thermal grounds. This includes endoscopic, transvaginal and transcutaneous applications.

Doppler

It has been demonstrated in experiments with unperfused tissue that some Doppler diagnostic equipment has the potential to produce biologi-cally significant temperature rises, specifically at bone/soft tissue interfaces. The effects of ele-vated temperatures may be minimized by keep-ing the time for which the beam passes through any one point in tissue as short as possible. Where output power can be controlled, the lowest available power level consistent with obtaining the desired diagnostic information should be used.

Although the data on humans are sparse, it is clear from animal studies that exposures result-ing in temperatures less than 38.5 °C can be used without reservation on thermal grounds. This includes obstetric applications.

Transducer heating

A substantial source of heating may be the trans-ducer itself. Tissue heating from this source is localized to the volume in contact with the trans-ducer.

CONCLUSIONS

Data from studies with rats demonstrate that exposure for 5 min to a temperature increase of 4 °C above the normal body temperature is haz-ardous to embryonic and fetal development. Similar thresholds have been reported for ultra-sound-induced heating of actively dividing cells in bone marrow. Temperature increases of approximately 4 °C have been measured, at or near bone/soft tissue interfaces in animal fetuses *in utero*, during exposure to conditions similar to those used in spectral pulsed Doppler diagnostic equipment.

The effects of elevated temperatures may be minimized by keeping the time for which the beam passes through any one point in tissue as short as possible.

The acoustic output from simple B-mode imaging is controlled to levels that are not capable of producing harmful temperature rises in tissue. Ultrasound scanning in B-mode is not contraindicated on thermal grounds.

References

1. NCRP (1992). *Exposure Criteria for Medical Diag-nostic Ultrasound: 1. Criteria Based on Thermal Mechanisms*, Report no. 113. (Bethesda, MD: National Council for Radiation Protection and Measurements)

2. Henderson, J., Willson, K., Jago, J. R. and Whit-tingham, T. A. (1995). A survey of the acoustic outputs of diagnostic ultrasound equipment in current clinical use. *Ultrasound Med. Biol.*, **21**, 699–705.

3. AIUM/NEMA (1992). *Standard for Real-Time Display of Thermal and Mechanical Acoustic Output Indices on Diagnostic Ultrasound Equipment.* (Rockville, MD: American Institute of Ultrasound in Medicine)

4. Bly, S. H. P., Vlahovich, S., Mabee, P. R. and Hussey, R. G. (1992). Computed estimates of maximum temperature elevations in fetal tissue during transabdominal pulsed Doppler examinations. *Ultrasound Med. Biol.*, **18**, 389–97

5. AIUM (1994). *Bioeffects and Safety of Diagnostic Ultrasound.* (Laurel, MD: American Institute of Ultrasound in Medicine)

6. Patton, C. A., Harris, G. R. and Phillips, R. A. (1994). Output levels and bioeffects indices from diagnostic ultrasound exposure data reported to the FDA. *IEEE Trans. UFFC,* **41**, 353–9

7. ter Haar, G. R., Duck, F. A., Starritt, H. C. and Daniels, S. (1989). Biophysical characterisation of diagnostic ultrasound equipment – preliminary results. *Phys. Med. Biol.*, **34**, 1533–42

8. WFUMB (1992). In Barnett, S. B. and Kossoff, G. (eds.) Issues and recommendations regarding thermal mechanisms for biological effects of ultrasound. World Federation for Ultrasound in Medicine and Biology Symposium on Safety and Standardisation in Medical Ultrasound. Special issue, No. 9. *Ultrasound Med. Biol.*, **18**

9. Bosward, K. L., Barnett, S. B., Wood, A. K. W., Edwards, M. J. and Kossoff, G. (1993). Heating of the guinea-pig fetal brain during exposure to pulsed ultrasound. *Ultrasound Med. Biol.*, **19**, 415–24

10. Horder, M. M., Barnett, S. B., Vella, G. and Edwards, M. J. (1997). Ultrasound-induced temperature increase in the guinea-pig fetal brain *in vitro*. *Ultrasound Med. Biol.*, in press

11. Drewniak, J. L., Carnes, K. I. and Dunn, F. (1989). *In vitro* ultrasound heating of fetal bone. *J. Acoust. Soc. Am.*, **88**, 26–34

12. Wu, J., Chase, J. D., Zhu, Z. and Holzapfel, T. F. (1992). Temperature rise in a tissue-mimicking material generated by unfocused and focused transducers. *Ultrasound Med. Biol.*, **18**, 495–512

13. O'Neill, T., Winkler, A. J. and Wu, J. (1994). Ultrasound heating in a tissue–bone phantom. *Ultrasound Med. Biol.*, **20**, 579–88

14. Wu, J., Cubberley, F., Gormley, G. and Szabo, T. L. (1995). Temperature rise generated by diagnostic ultrasound in a transcranial phantom. *Ultrasound Med. Biol.*, **21**, 561–8

15. Carstensen, E. L., Child, S. Z., Norton, S. and Nyborg, W. L. (1990). Ultrasonic heating of the skull. *J. Acoust. Soc. Am.*, **87**, 1310–17

16. Horder, M. M., Barnett, S. B., Edwards, M. J. and Kossoff, G. (1993). *In vivo* temperature rise in the fetus from duplex Doppler ultrasound. In

Proceedings of the 23rd Annual Conference of the Australasian Society of Ultrasound in Medicine, pp. 66, Melbourne, Australia, September, abstr.

17. Duggan, P. M., Liggins, G. C. and Barnett, S. B. (1995). Ultrasonic heating of the brain of the fetal sheep *in utero*. *Ultrasound Med. Biol.*, **21**, 553–60

18. Horder, M. M., Barnett, S. B., Vella, G., Edwards, M. J. and Wood, A. K. W. (1997). *In vivo* heating of the guinea-pig fetal brain during exposure to pulsed ultrasound. *Ultrasound Med. Biol.,* in press

19. Tarantal, A. F., Chu, F., O'Brien, W. D. and Hendrickx, A. G. (1993). Sonographic heat generation *in vivo* in the gravid long-tailed macaque (*Macaca fascicularis*). *J. Ultrasound Med.,* **5**, 285–95

20. Kimmel, G. L., Cuff, J. M., Kimmel, C. A., Heredia, D. J., Tudor, N., Silverman, P. M. and Chen, J. (1993). Skeletal development following heat exposure in the rat. *Teratology,* **47**, 229–42

21. Edwards, M. J., Mulley, R., Ring, S. and Wanner, R. A. (1974). Mitotic cell death and delay in mitotic activity in guinea-pig embryos following brief maternal hyperthermia. *J. Embryol Exp. Morph.,* **32**, 593–602

22. Upfold, J. B., Smith, M. S. R. and Edwards, M. J. (1989). Quantitative study of the effects of maternal hyperthermia on cell death and proliferation in the guinea-pig brain on day 21 of pregnancy. *Teratology,* **39**, 173–9

23. Edwards, M. J. (1993). Hyperthermia and birth defects. *Cornell Vet.,* **83**, 1–7

24. Miller, M. W. and Ziskin, M. C. (1989). Biological consequences of hyperthermia. *Ultrasound Med. Biol.,* **15**, 707–22

25. Barnett, S. B., ter Haar, G. R., Ziskin, M. C., Nyborg, W. L., Maeda, K. and Bang, J. (1994). Current status of research on biophysical effects of ultrasound. *Ultrasound Med. Biol.,* **20**, 205–18

26. Germain, M. A., Webster, W. S. and Edwards, M. J. (1985). Hyperthermia as a teratogen: parameters determining hyperthermia-induced head defects in the rat. *Teratology,* **31**, 265–72

27. Sasaki, J., Yamaguchi, A., Nabeshima, Y., Shigemitsu, S., Mesaki, N. and Kubo, T. (1995). Exercise at high temperature causes maternal hyperthermia and fetal anomalies in rats. *Teratology,* **51**, 233–6

28. Webster, W. S. and Edwards, M. J. (1984). Hyperthermia and the induction of neural tube defects in mice. *Teratology,* **29**, 417–25

29. Shiota, K. (1988). Induction of neural tube defects and skeletal malformations in mice following brief hyperthermia *in utero*. *Biol. Neonate,* **53**, 86–97

30. Edwards, M. J., Shiota, K., Smith, M. S. R. and Walsh, D. A. (1995). Hyperthermia and birth defects. *Reprod. Toxicol.,* **9**, 411–25

31. Edwards, M. J. and Penny, R. H. C. (1985). Effects of hyperthermia on the myelograms of adult and fetal guinea-pigs. *Br. J. Radiol.*, **59**, 93–101

32. Barnett, S. B., Edwards, M. J. and Martin, P. (1991). Pulsed ultrasound induces temperature elevation and nuclear abnormalities in bone marrow cells of guinea-pig femurs, abstr. 3405. *Proceedings of the 6th WFUMB Congress in Ultrasound*, Copenhagen, Denmark, September

33. Angles, J. M., Walsh, D. A., Li, K., Barnett, S. B. and Edwards, M. J. (1990). Effects of pulsed ultrasound and temperaure on the development of rat embryos in culture. *Teratology*, **42**, 285–93

34. Barnett, S. B., Walsh, D. A. and Angles, J. A. (1990). Novel approach to evaluate the interaction of pulsed ultrasound with embryonic development. *Ultrasonics*, **28**, 166–70

35. Wood, C. and Beard, R. W. (1964). Temperature of the human fetus. *J. Obstet. Gynaecol. Br. Commonwlth.*, **71**, 768–9

36. Walker, D., Walker, A. and Wood, C. (1969). Temperature of the human fetus. *J. Obstet. Gynaecol. Br. Commonwlth.*, **76**, 503–11

37. Bell, A. W. (1987). Consequences of severe heat stress for fetal development. In Hales, J. R. S. and Richards, D. A. B. (eds.) *Heat Stress: Physical Exertion and Environment.* (Amsterdam: Elsevier Science Publishers)

38. Edwards, M. J. (1986). Hyperthermia as a teratogen: a review of experimental studies and their clinical significance. *Teratogen. Carcinogen. Mutagen.*, **6**, 563–82

39. Erickson, J. D. (1991). Risk factors for birth defects: data from the Atlanta birth defects case–control study. *Teratology*, **43**, 41–51

40. Shepard, T. H. (1982). Detection of human teratogenic agents. *J. Pediatr.*, **101**, 810–15

41. Shepard, T. H. (1989). *Catalogue of Teratogenic Agents.* (Baltimore: Johns Hopkins University Press)

42. Smith, D. W., Clarren, S. K. and Harvey, M. A. S. (1978). Hyperthermia as a possible teratogenic agent. *J. Pediatr.*, **92**, 878–83

43. Layde, P. M., Edmonds, L. D. and Erickson, J. D. (1980). Maternal fever and neural tube defects. *Teratology*, **21**, 105–8

44. Pleet, H., Graham, J. M. and Smith, D. W. (1981). Central nervous system and facial defects associated with hyperthermia at four to 14 weeks gestation. *Paediatrics*, **67**, 785–9

45. Shiota, K. (1982). Neural tube defects and maternal hyperthermia in early pregnancy: epidemiology in a human embryo population. *Am. J. Med. Genet.*, **12**, 281–8

46. Spraggett, K. and Fraser, F. C. (1982). Teratogenicity of maternal fever in women; a retrospective study. *Teratology*, **25**, 75A

Effects of ultrasound exposure on fetal development in animal models

5

A. F. Tarantal

SUMMARY

The goal of this chapter is to provide a balanced view of current knowledge on the effects of diagnostic ultrasound on fetal development and to describe the developmental time points and organ systems that may be sensitive to exposure. From experimental evidence in relevant animal models, it has been shown that biological effects can occur during gestation. Studies on fetal growth have suggested the possibility of inducing growth-restrictive mechanisms in various animal models. It is proposed that growth factors such as insulin-like growth factor (IGF) and heat shock proteins (hsps) may be involved in this effect. Fetal hematopoietic changes during a defined period of development have also been well documented in a monkey model, although these findings were transient, with no long-term ramifications reported. The fetal brain and lung have also been proposed as possible areas of sensitivity; however, there has been little evidence to support a direct effect on either organ system.

INTRODUCTION

The frequency of use of diagnostic ultrasound in obstetrics has continued to rise as equipment design and sophisticated techniques for monitoring fetal development have evolved. Two-dimensional imaging techniques are routinely used for assessing growth and developmental anatomy, and pulsed and color Doppler are applied for monitoring uteroplacental and fetal blood flow under a variety of conditions. Although diagnostic ultrasound is reliable for obtaining essential information on fetal status, many gaps remain in our understanding of the interaction of this imaging modality with tissues, particularly during pregnancy. The fetus is a special case when safety issues are addressed, since the length of the examination period, scanning techniques chosen, equipment used for the examination, experience of the operator and gestational age are all known to affect the 'dose' received by the conceptus *in utero*[1].

The current general impression is that the clinical application of diagnostic ultrasound is 'safe' and poses no risk to the embryo or fetus. However, many questions remain regarding the interaction of ultrasound with developing tissues, because:

(1) Our knowledge of ultrasound-derived biological effects is incomplete;

(2) The extent of use of ultrasound during pregnancy continues to increase;

(3) Technological advances lead to increased acoustic power and enhanced potential for tissue interactions such as heating and cavitation;

(4) In the USA, limitations on the output intensity (spatial peak temporal average, I_{SPTA}) have increased for fetal applications; and

(5) Evidence of transient effects in humans[2,3] and in relevant animal models[4-7] have been reported at diagnostic exposure levels.

Although, to date, no long-term ramifications of prenatal diagnostic ultrasound exposure have been identified in either humans or mammalian models, it is essential that any evidence which suggests the possibility of an effect be explored, and the conditions which could enhance the likelihood of an interaction be known. The principal source of such data will be from experimental studies with animal models where investigations can be conducted under controlled conditions.

The intent of this chapter is to discuss fetal organ systems that are potentially sensitive to exposure to diagnostic ultrasound. Those areas of bioeffects investigation which have direct relevance to current human fetal scanning conditions and exposures will be described; however, this chapter is not intended to provide an exhaustive review of the bioeffect literature. Readers are referred to the many excellent reviews and society publications for further information[8-17], and to other chapters in this volume.

FETAL GROWTH

There have been reports that fetal and newborn body weights are lower than the normal range following ultrasound exposure in animal models[4-7] as well as in the human[2,3]. There are several reviews on this subject[11,13,15,18]. Although the mechanism whereby ultrasound can affect the growth process is currently unclear, reports of an association continue to appear. Intrauterine growth restriction (IUGR) frequently warrants repetitive sonographic evaluations in order to monitor growth progression and ultimate outcome. Therefore, if frequent ultrasound exposure can affect the growth process, this raises questions regarding its impact in general, and on the growth-compromised fetus in particular.

In vivo studies

Decreased fetal body weights after prenatal exposure to ultrasound have been reported in the mouse[19,20] and monkey[4-7], although this has not been a consistent finding in all species studied[19,21-24]. For example, studies with mice have shown significant dose-dependent effects on fetal weight (exposure from 10 to 300 s on gestational day (GD) 8; intensities ranged from 0.5 to 5.5 W/cm[2]), whereas mouse hybrids exposed under the same conditions in the same laboratory did not show a significant effect[19,25].

It was hypothesized that hybrid strains may be more resistant than outbred strains; however, a similar dose-dependent response was found by others (exposures on GD 1 to 13; 1 W/cm^2)[26]. In contrast, a study with pregnant rats exposed daily to continuous wave ultrasound (GD 4 to 19; 3 MHz, I_{SPTA} = 0.1-30 W/cm^2; 15 min duration per exposure) have shown no fetal growth-related effects when evaluated at term[24]. Another study[22] did not reveal any significant alterations in neonatal growth or development after exposure on GD 15, 17 and 19 (5.0 MHz, pulse repetition frequency (PRF) = 1 kHz, I_{SPTA}, 24 mW/cm^2).

Unlike studies with the rodent, investigations with the monkey have consistently shown transient reductions in body weights under various ultrasound imaging conditions (two-dimensional, pulsed Doppler, 'triple mode'). In a number of studies frequent exposure to clinically relevant levels of ultrasound have been performed during all stages of gestation (approximately 40 exposures)[4-7]. The original goals of these investigations were (1) to explore the potential long-term manifestations of frequent intrauterine exposure, and (2) to identify susceptible organ systems and gestational time points. Studies were conducted with standard two-dimensional (B-mode) imaging[4-6,27] in addition to 'triple mode' exposures (two-dimensional plus pulsed and color Doppler)[7]. For two-dimensional exposures, examinations were performed daily for 5 consecutive days each week from GD 21 to 35 (10 min per exposure; early first trimester), three times weekly from GD 36 to 60 (10 min per exposure; late first trimester), then weekly from GD 61 to term (20 min per exposure; second and third trimesters) ($n = 27$). Controls ($n = 25$) were 'scanned' with the unit placed on 'standby' during the same time intervals. Trimesters are divided by 55-day increments in this species, with pregnancy duration 165 ± 10 days. For triple mode, exposures ($n = 17$) were performed during GD 20 to 60 (five times weekly from GD 20 to 35, three times weekly from GD 36 to 60) for 5 min duration with the Doppler sample volume placed in the heart, and weekly from GD 61 to term for a total 10 min exposure

(5 min with the sample volume placed within the heart, 5 min within the umbilical cord at the abdominal insertion site; $n = 8$ sham controls). Fetal blood samples were collected in ketamine-sedated animals by ultrasound-guided cardiocentesis[28] on GD 120 and 140 (third trimester) and from the umbilical cord at birth. Simian Apgar scores and physical, morphometric and placental evaluations were performed at Cesarean section, as previously described[4,5], with multiple postnatal assessments for 4–6 months postnatal age thereafter (see further comments on growth, hematology and development, below). Body weights were typically decreased for most exposed animals at birth when compared to controls; however, all were within the control range within 3 months' postnatal age[5–7]. Therefore, all exposed animals showed 'catch-up' growth in the early postnatal period and were in the range of normal for body weight from 3 months onward.

Possible mechanisms: growth factors and heat shock proteins

Several fetal factors have been proposed to play a role in the growth-related effects observed as a result of chronic ultrasound exposure, although there is no current evidence that definitively explains these findings. One hypothesis is that tissue heating is the primary insult, with subsequent effects on the IGF axis and/or hsps[7]. The generation of heat during exposure to ultrasound is a well described phenomenon, with areas most likely to absorb ultrasonic energy being those directly associated with bone and at muscle/bone interfaces. The fetal skeleton is, therefore, important in this regard, since increasing ossification occurs during prenatal life. Tissue heating is discussed in Chapter 4; readers are referred to this chapter for further discussions on this topic.

IGF axis

Since the IGF axis (IGF-I, IGF-II, IGF binding proteins, IGF receptors) is known to play a central role in fetal growth[29–31], evaluations of these important mitogenic and differentiative factors have been proposed to provide important insights into bioeffects mechanisms[7]. Fetal growth is a complex process involving multiple factors; fetal IGF production is known to be essential[29,30]. Gene knock-out experiments have shown that loss of the IGF peptide or receptors may result in death of the conceptus in utero or postnatally, or in the severe IUGR associated with postnatal mortality. In the mammalian fetus, circulating concentrations of IGF increase during gestation[32–34], although little free (unbound) IGF is in the circulation, owing to high concentrations of IGF binding proteins (IGFBPs)[35,36]. The functions of the IGFBPs include: (1) increasing the circulating half-life of IGF; (2) transporting the IGFs (IGF-I, IGF-II) in the circulation and within the vascular compartments; (3) localizing the IGFs to specific cell types; and (4) modulating growth-promoting actions. The interaction between IGFs and the predominant circulating IGFBP, IGFBP-3, is a delicate balance between the inhibitory or potentiating effects of soluble IGFBP-3 vs. cell-associated IGFBP-3[35]. The IGFBPs display a high and specific affinity for IGF. Since IGFBPs can associate with cell membranes and elements of the extracellular matrix, it has been proposed that a partitioning of available IGFs between the IGF receptor and membrane-bound, matrix-bound, or soluble IGFBPs is a potential mechanism for regulating IGF bioavailability[35]. IGFBP-3, for example, has been proposed to have a different affinity for IGF-I in fluids vs. a membrane-bound state. Further, evidence that the IGFBPs facilitate the translocation of IGFs across endothelial boundaries supports an endocrine role for the IGFs, while the expression of the IGFs and the type 1 IGF receptor in fetal tissues suggests that actions are also exerted locally, either on cells of synthesis (an autocrine action) or those in close proximity (a paracrine role). Experimental findings have suggested that, although many fetal cells may possess IGF receptors and are responsive to exogenous IGF, they are not necessarily capable of synthesis[37–40].

In both the human[33] and non-human[34] fetal primate, serum IGF-I and IGF-II levels increase with advancing gestation, and alterations in this developmental profile have been correlated with abnormal growth patterns[33]. Studies with fetal monkeys frequently exposed to ultrasound and blood sampled periodically during gestation have shown aberrations in the IGF axis[7]. Here, a transient elevation in IGF-I and a significant reduction in circulating IGFBP-3 was shown. The reduction in circulating IGFBP-3 may be a compensatory response which protects the ultrasound-exposed fetus from severe growth alterations. Thus, monkey fetuses were small-for-gestational-age at birth, but not severely growth restricted. The direct mechanism(s) for effects on the IGF axis are currently unclear, and will require further investigation.

It is important to note that growth factors such as the IGFs and cytokines such as tumor necrosis factor-α (TNF-α) and the interleukins (IL) form a large family of extracellular signalling molecules with very similar mechanisms of action on fetal growth. For example, a role for TNF-α in IUGR has been proposed[41], and interactions between the IGFs and TNF-α involving local IGFBP regulation have been shown[42]. TNF-α has been reported to alter the endocrine action of the IGFs by interacting with IGFBP-3 secretion; this could imply an important role for TNF-α during chronic ultrasound exposure. Thermal stimulation and/or inflammatory changes can set in motion a series of events promoting production of synergistic cytokines such as TNF-α and interleukins (IL-1, IL-6), as well as growth factors such as the IGFs. IL-6 can function as a 'hepatocyte stimulating factor' and, with IL-1 and TNF-α, is a primary inducer of the hepatic acute-phase response, a cell defence mechanism initiated after organ injury; human fetal liver cells have shown the capacity to elicit this response[43]. Since immunocytochemical studies have identified the fetal liver as a major site of IGF and IGFBP production[37–39], ultrasound-induced hepatic heating may be a significant event. This hypothesis is supported by preliminary evidence in the monkey, in which frequent, acute fetal temperature elevations of 2.5 °C produce a similar effect on growth and the IGF axis, as observed with chronic ultrasound exposure (A. F. Tarantal, unpublished). More studies will, however, be required in order to support these hypotheses.

Heat shock proteins (Hsps) and thermotolerance

In addition to the potential role of the IGF axis, it is also possible that hsps, or 'stress proteins', may participate in modifying the growth-related effects observed in fetuses exposed to ultrasound, and could explain the variation reported in individual studies. Hsps represent a cellular defense mechanism following stressors such as heat shock, inflammation, fever, viral infection, or anoxia[44]. Hsps have been studied for their physiological significance in the maintenance of cellular integrity, and many of these proteins have been shown to participate in essential metabolic processes and to regulate cell growth and differentiation. Hsps are typically named and classified in different families according to molecular mass (e.g. hsp 70, hsp 90).

In all cells and organisms, mild heat shocks can induce an increase in thermoresistance to subsequent hyperthermic exposures[44]. When exposed to non-lethal heat shock, mammalian cells can acquire a transient resistance to subsequent exposures at elevated temperatures, thereby developing thermotolerance. Thus, hsps may provide some degree of thermotolerance and protection as a result of heating during ultrasound exposure, as reported under other experimental conditions[45]. Little information is currently available on the generation of hsps in the fetus *in vivo*[46,47], particularly in response to ultrasound exposure[48]. It is also not known whether repeated, incremental thermal exposures of short duration such as with ultrasound exposure can result in a protective mechanism such as thermotolerance, and whether a critical threshold exists whereby a switch from a protective to a potentially detrimental effect can occur[49–51]. Although reports have suggested that a rise of at least 2.0 °C over baseline temperature must occur for effects on cell viability or cyclicity, it has not been established that elevations of ≤ 1.0 °C do not result in a biological effect that is significant. More studies in these areas will be required in order to elucidate the role of hsps and thermotolerance in growth-regulating mechanisms and the relationship to ultrasound exposure.

FETAL HEMATOPOIESIS

Multiple bioeffect investigations have focused on various hematological aspects such as hemolysis, platelets and coagulation, and neutrophil and lymphocyte production and function in adult and fetal models both *in vitro* and *in vivo*[40–47,52–54]. Readers are referred to reviews on these topics[54]; only studies with direct relevance to the human fetus are discussed below.

Hematopoietic ontogeny

In order to understand the potential impact ultrasound can have on hematopoiesis (blood cell formation) during fetal life, it is important to review essential developmental events. Fetal hematopoiesis involves multiple compartments, with blood cell formation a consequence of hematopoietic stem cell (HSC) migration and seeding[55]. The initial source of HSC is the extra-embryonic mesenchyme of the yolk sac wall and associated structures, with stem and erythropoietic cells migrating from these sites to the embryonic circulation, beginning roughly in the 4th week of gestation. Migration of HSC into the hepatic primordia for establishment of hematopoiesis occurs during weeks 5–6 of (human) pregnancy[55]. The liver becomes the major source of blood cells, with a peak in production at the 3rd month, and subsequent decline after the 7th month of pregnancy. The bone marrow becomes an active site of hematopoiesis at 10–11 weeks' gestation. Bone marrow hematopoiesis is initiated with immigration of the vascularized mesenchyme into cavities left by decaying cartilage, and stromal matrix develops approximately 2 weeks prior to accepting the immigration of blood-borne HSC.

Fetal liver remains hematopoietic during fetal life and the first postnatal week, although the magnitude of its hematopoietic activity is considerably reduced during this stage of development. Hematopoiesis in the liver is predominantly erythropoietic, with fewer granulocytes and lymphocytes present[55]. Human fetuses do, however, have a substantial fraction of neutrophil reserves within liver and spleen; at term, the liver still contains roughly 60–70% of this reserve, although by 2 weeks' postnatal age the marrow contains essentially all of the stored neutrophils[56].

Comparable hematopoietic events occur in the monkey at developmental time periods similar to those of humans[28] (A. F. Tarantal, unpublished). The liver is the primary site of hematopoiesis during the late first trimester in the fetal monkey (approximately GD 45–50; comparable to weeks 5–6 in the human), with a peak in hepatic hematopoiesis shortly thereafter (roughly 3–4 months in the human). The source of blood cell formation changes from the liver to the bone marrow as a gradual process, occurring over an extended period during the second and third trimesters in both species. Comparable to the human fetus, during this time both organs are a hematopoietic source. Early signs of bone marrow hematopoiesis occur in the fetal monkey during the early second trimester, similar to the human. Therefore, the monkey provides an excellent model for studying the hematopoietic effects of ultrasound exposure *in utero*.

In vivo studies

Studies in fetal mice have shown that exposures at varying intensities (0.1–3.0 W/cm^2) and gestational ages do not effect lymphocyte development or function[52,53]. Although studies with fetal monkeys chronically exposed to ultrasound at diagnostic levels (see discussion under Fetal growth, above), and sampled periodically *in utero*, have also shown no effects on lymphocyte counts, significant effects on the neutrophil lineage have been consistently observed during the third trimester[5–7]. Under all imaging conditions studied (two-dimensional, triple mode), neutrophil counts were marginally reduced on GD 120 (early third trimester), significantly diminished on GD 140 (mid-third trimester), and elevated at term, with a return to the control range in the postnatal period. When fetal blood was grown in culture, progenitor assays revealed significant reductions in the colony forming unit-granulocyte–macrophage (CFU-GM), the hematopoietic progenitor cell responsible for granulocyte and macrophage production, on all days evaluated (GD 120, 140, term)[7]. Aspirates of bone marrow collected on the day of delivery showed exuberant growth for exposed animals, with cell counts comparable to controls. Postnatal evaluations indicated an elevation of CFU-GM growth during the 1st week of life, with a return to control values by 1 month postnatal age. The effects on the neutrophil lineage occurred after chronic and frequent 20-min exposures to two-dimensional (B-mode) imaging or 10-min exposures to triple mode, where the thermal elevations at each exposure were approximately 1 °C[57]. These data suggest an inability of the progenitor population to enter the fetal circulation, although the precise mechanism for these findings will require further investigation.

Possible mechanisms: cell death, adhesion, and margination

Effective hematopoiesis is a multi-step process consisting of HSC proliferation and cell maintenance, differentiation into committed cell populations, orderly maturation into functional cells and transport into the circulation, depending on body demands. Within this cascade of events are potential explanations for the hematopoietic changes observed in third-trimester monkey fetuses chronically exposed to ultrasound *in utero*. There may be a transient decrease in production of the CFU-GM, defective maturation of this differentiated population, or sequestration of cells within the hematopoietic tissues (liver and/or bone marrow). Any of these changes could affect both mature (neutrophil) and immature (CFU-GM) cell populations in the peripheral circulation. Elevated CFU-GM in the bone marrow at term in fetal monkeys is suggestive of bone marrow pooling, although these findings could represent a compensatory response, particularly as the bone marrow takes on a more central hematopoietic role.

Three factors can influence blood neutrophil concentration. These include the rate of input from the bone marrow storage pool and the liver to the blood, the proportion of cells circulating compared with marginated (adhered to or rolling along the vessel wall), and the rate at which cells are leaving the blood. Under some conditions, and as a result of inflammation or altered hemodynamics, perhaps as a result of tissue heating, ultrasound exposure may induce cell adhesion, with a subsequent shift in the population from the circulating to the marginated pool. Transient hemodynamic changes have been shown to induce a 'pseudoneutropenia' with an increased proportion of cells in the peripheral blood as marginated vs. freely circulating. Under these circumstances, peripheral blood cell counts would not accurately reflect the total number of blood cells present. Neutrophils constitutively express cell adhesion molecules and can rapidly alter their number or functional state in response to specific stimuli[58]. This process can be rapidly reversed or even sustained for hours, depending upon the nature of the stimulus.

Based on current experimental evidence it has been proposed that an increase in cell adhesion occurs in the fetal circulation as a result of ultrasound exposure, with the primary insult hypothesized to be heating[7]. Because other laboratories have shown that CFU-GM are uniquely sensitive to heat when compared to other hematopoietic progenitor populations[59–61], it is also possible that peripheral cell killing occurs at the time of exposure. However, this is not supported by current *in vivo* evidence, and, therefore, margination is a more likely explanation[7]. To date, there have been no reports that have suggested similar hematopoietic effects in the human fetus. However, this may be due to the fact that effects are transient, there is limited sampling of fetuses (blood, bone marrow) during the periods identified as susceptible and no significant changes would be anticipated postnatally. It is important to note that, to date, all monkeys studied under all exposure conditions have resumed a normal postnatal developmental course, with no long-term hematological or health-related effects detected.

FETAL BRAIN

It has been well described that ultrasound has a selective capacity to interact with white vs. gray matter at high intensity levels[62], and that low-intensity effects on myelination can occur from both a structural and a functional perspective[63-67]. Heating has been reported to be one of the primary mechanisms responsible for these effects; the sensitivity of the central nervous system (CNS) to heat has been previously documented[13,68] (see Chapter 4). Although the fetal brain is clearly an organ that could be susceptible to the effects of ultrasound exposure, there are few studies which have addressed this topic in the fetus that are clinically relevant. However, owing to current knowledge regarding ultrasound-induced interactions with the brain under extreme conditions, the known frequency of exposure of the fetal and neonatal brain to ultrasound and our current understanding regarding normal neurodevelopmental processes, the fetal brain is worthy of discussion as an organ of potential susceptibility.

Neurodevelopment: myelination and neurogenesis

Myelination begins in the human fetus during the second trimester, although a significant degree of myelination continues after birth[69]. In humans, rapid myelination is well under way in the pons, medulla and structures formed from the mesencephalon by 20–30 weeks' gestation, whereas myelination begins at roughly 30–40 weeks' in structures within the forebrain. The time of onset varies for each mammalian species[69]. For example, the end of the most rapid phase of myelination is at 25 to 30 postnatal days in the rat as compared to 2 years of postnatal age in the human. The period of maximum vulnerability of myelination in the human corresponds with the time of the major growth spurt of the brain; from the 7th month of prenatal life through the first few months of postnatal age[70].

There is a close interdependency between myelination and neurogenesis. Neurogenesis occurs over a long developmental period with different neurons forming at different time points, and production declining as birth approaches[71]. Production periods can be as brief in species with long (human and non-human primates) as well as short (rodent) gesta-

tions. Many cells that form in late gestation in the mouse will form before mid-gestation in the monkey[72], although a period of postnatal proliferation is characteristic of both monkeys and humans[73-75]. Neurogenesis is virtually complete by the end of the 3rd week of human postnatal life. The degree of functional maturity at birth differs from species to species, with the human more advanced than the mouse or rat, and less advanced than the monkey[71]. Therefore, experimental studies that focus on the effects of ultrasound on brain development must take into account the differing time points at which particular developmental events take place, in order to maintain relevance to the human fetus.

Ex utero studies

Functional effects of low-intensity ultrasound have been reported in the neonatal rat[76]. Neonates of 3–5 days of age, which are roughly comparable to a third-trimester human fetus, were scanned for 30 min using a diagnostic system with an $I_{SPTA} = 0.135$ mW/cm^2 (3.5 MHz). Electron microscopy of sections of dorsal nerve roots post-exposure indicated a disruption of the nodes of Ranvier and morphological changes ranging from vacuole formation in the paranodal regions to frank demyelination. Although similar effects would not be anticipated under current in utero scanning conditions, these findings emphasize the potential sensitivity of the brain to ultrasound exposure at defined developmental periods.

In utero studies

Studies have been conducted with chronically instrumented fetal lambs during the third trimester[77]. Fetuses were exposed to a commercial scanner ($I_{SPTA} = 15.5$ mW/cm^2) for 15 min in order to evaluate the auditory brain stem response during exposure. A consistent decrease in the mean amplitude and an increase in the mean latency of all five wave deflections of the auditory brainstem response was observed. This effect appeared to be transitory, since all values approached baseline 30 min after cessation of ultrasound exposure. It was concluded that direct exposure of the fetal sheep brain *in vivo* may temporarily influence nerve conduction along CNS axonal pathways. Further studies with the sheep have focused on the effect of low intensity pulsed ultrasound on electrocortical activity[78]. Here, transducers generating 60 mW of power were attached to the fetal skull and impulses activated periodically of 30-s duration. Analysis of continuous recordings of electrocortical activity in this model showed no effects of exposure to pulsed ultrasound at intensity levels equivalent to those of standard two-dimensional imaging.

Others have evaluated the effects of heat on cerebral tissue after exposure of rodent embryos (via exteriorized uterine horns) to 43 °C for 8 min[79]. After growth in culture, no morphological differences were observed between control and exposed cerebral specimens, although a reduction in select enzymes (acetylcholinesterase (AchE) and 2′,3′-cyclic nucleotide phosphohydrolase (CNPase) was observed when compared to controls. These data were interpreted as an impairment in the development of neurons and oligodendrocytes, since AchE was used as a marker for cholinergic neurons and CNPase as a marker for oligodendrocytes and myelination. Follow-up studies examined the activities of these same biochemical markers[80]. Rat embryos (GD 10) were exposed in a similar manner to 5-min continuous wave ultrasound (2.5 W/cm^2; I$_{SATA}$ 1 MHz). Although no differences in brain weight or protein content were observed, a transient decrease in AchE and CNPase was noted in exposed specimens. Because of the exposure conditions, intensity levels, volume of tissue exposed and methods of exposure, the authors concluded that a similar event was unlikely to occur in the human clinical setting. Although other studies have reported enhancement of the neurotransmitters acetylcholine (ACh), γ-amino butyric acid (GABA), and AChE in exposed fetal mouse brains (continuous wave, 875 kHz, 1 W/cm^2 for 300–400 s over a 5-day period)[81], the relevance of these findings to the human fetus currently remains speculative.

Since it has been proposed that structural alterations of the brain can manifest as neuro-behavioral changes later in life, postnatal testing regimens have been used to evaluate postnatal outcome in humans as well as animal models such as rodents[15,22,24] and monkeys[5–7]. These studies have not provided conclusive evidence of any long-term ramifications of prenatal ultrasound exposure as it relates to neurological function or neurobehavioural development.

FETAL LUNG

An important question that needs to be fully examined is whether or not diagnostic pulsed ultrasound can alter fetal lung development. This has become a topic of interest, because lung lesions have been consistently produced in a range of mammalian species following exposure to diagnostic levels of ultrasound[17]. There is solid evidence that this effect results from the exposure of the lung, but it is not entirely clear what physical mechanism is the cause, although current theories propose it to be non-thermal. The essential element is the tissue/gas interface which appears to be required for a cavitation-related effect[17]. One study has reported the detection of inertial cavitation *in vivo* using the same diagnostic equipment that produced lung hemorrhage in rats[82].

The important question is: can a similar effect occur during fetal ultrasound exposure? Because future air spaces are extremely small and surrounded by rigid tissue boundaries, there is the potential for cellular injury (A. F. Tarantal, unpublished), should inertial cavitation occur. Since the fetal lung is fluid-filled for the entire period of gestation, this has been proposed to be unlikely. However, although there is no current evidence of damage to fetal lungs as a result of exposure to diagnostic ultrasound, it is possible that the third-trimester fetus and the neonate may be susceptible to cavitation-related[83] or other non-thermal effects. A recent study has demonstrated hemorrhage in fetal mouse tissues in close proximity to bone, including the lungs, after exposure to low-pressure amplitude lithotripter pulses[84]. The mechanism appears to be non-thermal and may be related to radiation pressure (see Chapter 9).

Since current clinical scanners have the capability of achieving high peak rarefactional pressures (see Chapter 3), and because there is an increased use of echocardiography in third-trimester fetuses and neonates with unavoidable exposure of lung, the possible occurrence of this phenomenon *in vivo* needs to be considered and assessed. Although, to date, there is no evidence to support the hypothesis that an effect on fetal lung can occur as a result of ultrasound exposure, it is a possibility that should be considered, because (1) damage that occurs may be repaired; (2) the most frequently scanned fetuses are those already compromised by a pre-existing disease (which would obscure the cause of damage); and (3) there is currently no information regarding the form that the injury would take.

The theoretical basis for the generation of cavitation nuclei in the fetus arises from bubble formation in lung tissue as the intra-alveolar surface tension changes, owing to the formation of surfactant, with bubble activity and growth enhanced once a negative pressure such as that supplied by ultrasound occurs. During the third trimester, a number of critical events occur in the fetal lung[85]. The gas exchange area (cuboidal epithelial lining) differentiates into two cell types, namely the alveolar type I and the type II cells. Active cell division occurs in both cell types, particularly in the type II population, which is responsible for active synthesis and secretion of pulmonary surfactant. This cuboidal population also undergoes squamation and migration in order to cover the potential air space surfaces and to fill a portion of the blood–air barrier. Both the differentiation of the type II cell biosynthetic and secretory capability and the squamation of type I cells are critical events for the formation of a respiratory system that provides respiratory gases after parturition. The impact which sequential injury could have on these two cell populations, and the effect this potential injury would have on further growth

and differentiation of the lung postnatally, have not been investigated.

CONCLUSIONS

Although studies performed, to date, have provided some degree of comfort regarding the safety of use of diagnostic ultrasound during pregnancy, our knowledge is clearly incomplete at this time. It is, therefore, important to note that the Food and Drug Administration, which regulates the output of radiological devices used in the USA, has recently revised its limitations on acoustic output of clinical scanners in an effort to eliminate imaging constraints on clinicians. Thus, the option for using additional acoustic power to obtain clinically useful information is available, which implies that a greater potential for biological interactions can occur as this power is increased. On-screen labelling has been developed to provide a means of indicating the relative risk of producing in tissue either a significant temperature increase (the thermal index, TI) or cavitation events (the mechanical index, MI)[86]. It is essential that users are knowledgable regarding the application of these indices, the capabilities of the systems with which they are scanning and methods for obtaining the required diagnostic information under the safest imaging conditions possible. With this goal in mind, ultrasound should remain a safe imaging modality for use during pregnancy. In the meantime, further mechanism-related investigations will be required in order to provide greater insight into conditions that increase the likelihood of a biological effect. It is important that these studies are continued using appropriate animal models with clinically relevant diagnostic equipment and exposure conditions. The continued prudent use of diagnostic ultrasound is warranted, and following the ALARA (as low as reasonably achievable) principle is essential.

References

1. Tarantal, A. F. and O'Brien, W. D. (1994). Discussion of ultrasonic safety related to obstetrics. In Sabbagha, R. E. (ed.) *Ultrasound Applied to Obstetrics and Gynecology*, 3rd edn, pp. 45–56. (Philadelphia: J. B. Lippincott)
2. Evans, S., Newnham, J., MacDonald, W. and Hall, C. (1996). Characterisation of the possible effect on birth weight following frequent prenatal ultrasound examinations. *Early Hum. Dev.*, **45**, 203–14
3. Newnham, J.P., Evans, S.F., Michael, C.A., Stanley, F.J. and Landau, L.I. (1993). Effects of frequent ultrasound during pregnancy: a randomised controlled trial. *Lancet*, **342**, 887–91
4. Tarantal, A. F. and Hendrickx, A. G. (1989). Evaluation of the bioeffects of prenatal ultrasound exposure in the cynomolgus macaque (*Macaca fascicularis*): I. Neonatal/infant observations. *Teratology*, **39**, 137–47
5. Tarantal, A. F. and Hendrickx, A. G. (1989). Evaluation of the bioeffects of prenatal ultrasound exposure in the cynomolgus macaque (*Macaca fascicularis*): II. Growth and behavior during the first year. *Teratology*, **39**, 149–62
6. Tarantal, A. F., O'Brien, W. D. and Hendrickx, A. G. (1993). Evaluation of the bioeffects of prenatal ultrasound exposure in the cynomolgus macaque (*Macaca fascicularis*): III. Developmental and hematologic studies. *Teratology*, **47**, 159–70
7. Tarantal, A. F., Gargosky, S. E., O'Brien, W. D. and Hendrickx, A. G. (1995). Haematologic and growth-related effects of frequent ultrasound exposure on fetal macaques (*Macaca fascicularis*). *Ultrasound Med. Biol.*, **21**, 1073–81
8. American Institute of Ultrasound in Medicine (AIUM) (1993). *Bioeffects and Safety of Diagnostic Ultrasound*. (Bethesda, MD: AIUM)
9. American Institute of Ultrasound in Medicine (AIUM) (1994). *Medical Ultrasound Safety*. (Bethesda, MD: AIUM)
10. Barnett, S. B., Ter Haar, G. R., Ziskin, M. C., Nyborg, W. L., Maeda, K. and Bang, J. (1994). Current status of research on biophysical effects of ultrasound. *Ultrasound Med. Biol.*, **20**, 205–18
11. Brent, R. L., Jensh, R. P. and Beckman, D. A. (1991). Medical sonography: reproductive effects and risks. *Teratology*, **44**, 123–46.
12. National Council on Radiation Protection and Measurements (NCRP) (1983). *Biological Effects of Ultrasound: Mechanisms and Clinical Implications*, Report no. 74. (Bethesda, MD: NCRP)
13. National Council on Radiation Protection and Measurements (NCRP) (1992). *Exposure Criteria for Medical Diagnostic Ultrasound: I. Criteria Based on Thermal Mechanisms*, Report no. 113. (Bethesda, MD: NCRP)
14. Nyborg, W. L. and Ziskin, M. C. (1985). *Biological Effects of Ultrasound*, Clinics in Diagnostic Ultrasound no. 16. (New York: Churchill Livingstone)
15. Stewart, H. D., Stewart, H. F., Moore, R. M. and Garry, J. (1985). Compilation of reported biological effects data and ultrasound exposure levels. *J. Clin. Ultrasound*, **13**, 167–86
16. Barnett, S. B. and Kossoff, G. (eds.) (1992). Issues and recommendations regarding thermal mechanisms for biological effects of ultrasound. In World Federation for Ultrasound in Medicine and Biology Symposium on Safety and Standardisation in Medical Ultrasound. *Ultrasound Med. Biol.*, **18**, Special Issue No.9
17. Barnett, S. B. (ed.) (1997). Conclusions and recommendations on thermal and non-thermal mechanisms for biological effects of ultrasound. In World Federation for Ultrasound in Medicine and Biology Symposium on Safety of Ultrasound in Medicine. *Ultrasound Med. Biol.*, in press
18. Miller, M. W. and Ziskin, M. C. (1989). Biological consequences of hyperthermia. *Ultrasound Med. Biol.*, **15**, 707–22
19. O'Brien, W. D. (1983). Dose-dependent effect of ultrasound on fetal weight in mice. *J. Ultrasound Med.*, **2**, 1–8
20. Hande, M. P. and Devi, P. U. (1993). Effect of *in utero* exposure to diagnostic ultrasound on the postnatal survival and growth of mouse. *Teratology*, **48**, 405–11
21. Child, S. Z., Hoffman, D., Strassner, D., Carstensen, E. L., Gates, A. H., Cox, C. and Miller, M. W. (1989). A test of I^2t as a dose parameter for fetal weight reduction from exposure to ultrasound. *Ultrasound Med. Biol.*, **15**, 39–44
22. Jensh, R. P., Lewin, P. A., Poczobutt, M. T., Goldberg, B. B., Oler, J. and Brent, R. L. (1994). The effects of prenatal ultrasound exposure on postnatal growth and acquisition of reflexes. *Radiat. Res.*, **140**, 284–93
23. Kimmel, C. A., Stratmeyer, M. E., Galloway, W. D., Brown, N. T., Laborder, J. B. and Bates, H. K. (1989). Developmental exposure of mice to pulsed ultrasound. *Teratology*, **40**, 387–93
24. Vorhees, C. V., Acuff-Smith, K. D., Weisenburger, W. P., Meyer, R. A., Smith, N. B. and O'Brien, W. D. Jr (1991). A teratologic evaluation of continuous-wave, daily ultrasound exposure in unanesthetized pregnant rats. *Teratology*, **44**, 667–74

25. O'Brien, W. D., Januzik, S. J. and Dunn, F. (1982). Ultrasound biologic effects: a suggestion of strain specificity. *J. Ultrasound Med.*, **1**, 367–70

26. Stolzenberg, S. J., Torbit, C. A., Pryor, G. T. and Edmonds, P. D. (1980). Toxicity of ultrasound in mice: neonatal studies. *Radiat. Environ. Biophys.*, **18**, 37–44

27. Tarantal, A. F. and Hendrickx, A. G. (1990). The effects of exposure of the macaque conceptus to ultrasound during organogenesis. *Am. J. Primatol.*, **20**, 237

28. Tarantal, A. F. (1993). Hematologic reference values for the fetal long-tailed macaque (*Macaca fascicularis*). *Am. J. Primatol.*, **29**, 209–19

29. DeChiara, T. M., Efstratiadis, A. and Robertson, E. J. (1990). A growth-deficiency phenotype in heterozygous mice carrying an insulin-like growth factor II gene disrupted by targeting. *Nature (London)*, **345**, 78–80

30. Liu, J.-P., Baker, J., Perkins, A. S., Robertson, E. J. and Efstratiadis, A. (1993). Mice carrying null mutations of the genes encoding insulin-like growth factor 1 (*Igf-1*) and type 1 IGF receptor (*Igf1r*). *Cell*, **75**, 59–72

31. Stewart, C. E. H. and Rotwein, P. (1996). Growth, differentiation and survival: multiple physiological functions for insulin-like growth factors. *Physiol. Rev.*, **76**, 1005–25

32. Chard, T. (1994). Insulin-like growth factors and their binding proteins in normal and abnormal human fetal growth. *Growth Regul.*, **4**, 91–100

33. Giudice, L. C., deZegher, F., Gargosky, S. E., Dsupin, B. A., de las Fuentas, L., Crystal, R. A., Hintz, R. L. and Rosenfeld, R. G. (1995). Insulin-like growth factors and their binding proteins in the term and pre-term human fetus and neonate with normal and extremes of intra-uterine growth. *J. Clin. Endocrinol. Metab.*, **80**, 1548–55

34. Tarantal, A. F. and Gargosky, S. E. (1995). Characterization of the insulin-like growth factor (IGF) axis in the serum of maternal and fetal macaques (*Macaca mulatta* and *Macaca fascicularis*). *Growth Regul.*, **5**, 190–8

35. Clemmons, D. R. (1993). IGF binding proteins and their functions. *Molec. Reprod. Dev.*, **35**, 368–75

36. Jones, J. and Clemmons, D. R. (1995). Insulin-like growth factors and their binding proteins: biological actions. *Endocr. Rev.*, **16**, 3–34

37. Han, V. K. M., D'Ercole, A. J. and Lund, P. K. (1987). Cellular localization of somatomedin (insulin-like growth factor) messenger RNA in the human fetus. *Science*, **236**, 193–7

38. Han, V. K. M., Hill, D. J., Strain, A. J., Towle, A. C., Lauder, J. M., Underwood, L. E. and D'Ercole, A. J. (1987). Identification of somatomedin/insulin-like growth factor immuno-reactive cells in the human fetus. *Pediatr. Res.*, **22**, 245–9

39. Han, V. K. M., Lund, P. K., Lee, D. C. and D'Ercole, A. J. (1988). Expression of somatomedin/IGF mRNAs in the human fetus: identification, characterization, and tissue distribution. *J. Clin. Endocrinol. Metab.*, **66**, 422–9

40. Han, V. K. M., Matsell, D. G., Delhanty, P. J. D., Hill, D. J., Shimasaki, S. and Nygard, K. (1996). IGF-binding protein mRNAs in the human fetus: tissue and cellular distribution of developmental expression. *Horm. Res.*, **45**, 160–6

41. Schiff, E., Friedman, S. A., Baumann, P., Sibai, B. M. and Romero, R. (1994). Tumor necrosis factor-α in pregnancies associated with pre-eclampsia or small-for-gestational-age newborns. *Am. J. Obstet. Gynecol.*, **170**, 1224–9

42. Yateman, M. E., Claffey, D. C., Cwyfan-Hughes, S. C., Frost, V. J., Wass, J. A. H. and Holly, J. M. P. (1993). Cytokines modulate the sensitivity of human fibroblasts to stimulation with insulin-like growth factor-I (IGF-I) by altering endogenous IGF-binding protein production. *J. Endocrinol.*, **137**, 151–9

43. Bauer, J., Lengyel, G., Thung, S. N., Jonas, U., Gerok, W. and Acs, G. (1991). Human fetal hepatocytes respond to inflammatory mediators and excrete bile. *Hepatology*, **13**, 1131–41

44. Li, G. C., Mivechi, N. F. and Weitzel, G. (1995). Heat shock proteins, thermotolerance, and their relevance to clinical hyperthermia. *Int. J. Hypertherm.*, **11**, 459–88

45. Burdon, R. H. (1986). Heat shock and the heat shock proteins. *Biochem. J.*, **240**, 313–24

46. Brown, I. R. (1983). Hyperthermia induces the synthesis of a heat shock protein by polysomes isolated from the fetal and neonatal mammalian brain. *J. Neurochem.*, **40**, 1490–3

47. White, F. P. (1981). The induction of 'stress' proteins in organ slices from brain, heart, and lung as a function of postnatal development. *J. Neurol.*, **1**, 1311–19

48. Angles, J. M., Walsh, D. A., Li, K., Barnett, S. B. and Edwards, M. J. (1990). Effects of pulsed ultrasound and temperature on the development of rat embryos in culture. *Teratology*, **42**, 285–93

49. Bennett, G. D., Mohl, V. K. and Finnell, R. H. (1990). Embryonic and maternal heat shock responses to a teratogenic hyperthermic insult. *Reprod. Tox.*, **4**, 113–19

50. German, J. (1984). Embryonic stress hypothesis of teratogenesis. *Am. J. Med.*, **76**, 293–301

51. Gericke, G. S., Hofmeyr, G. J., Laburn, H. and Isaacs, H. (1989). Does heat damage fetuses? *Med. Hypoth.*, **29**, 275–8

52. Desai, B. B., Sosolik, R. C., Ciaravino, V. and Teale, J. M. (1989). Effect of fetal exposure to

ultrasound on the development of functional, antigen-specific B lymphocytes in fetal and neonatal BALB/c mice. *Ultrasound Med. Biol.,* **15**, 575–80

53. Sosolik, R. C., Desai, B. B., Ciaravino, V. and Teale, J. M. (1989). Effect of fetal exposure to ultrasound on B lymphocyte function and antibody class production. *Ultrasound Med. Biol.,* **15**, 581–7

54. Williams, A. R. (1985). Effects of ultrasound on blood and the circulation. In Nyborg, W. L. and Ziskin, M. C. (eds.) *Biological Effects of Ultrasound,* Clinics in Diagnostic Ultrasound no. 16, pp. 49–65 (New York: Churchill Livingstone)

55. Kelemen, E., Calvo, W. and Fliedner, T. M. (1979). *Atlas of Human Hemopoietic Development.* (New York: Springer-Verlag)

56. Christensen, R. D. (1989). Haematopoiesis in the fetus and neonate. *Pediatr. Res.,* **26**, 531–5

57. Tarantal, A. F., Chu, F., O'Brien, W. D. and Hendrickx, A. G. (1993). Sonographic heat generation *in vivo* in the gravid long-tailed macaque (*Macaca fascicularis*). *J. Ultrasound Med.,* **12**, 285–95

58. Zimmerman, G. A., Prescott, S. M. and McIntyre, T. M. (1992). Endothelial cell interactions with granulocytes: tethering and signaling molecules. *Immunol. Today,* **13**, 93–100

59. Mivechi, N. F. (1988). Heat sensitivity, thermotolerance and profile of protein synthesis of human bone marrow progenitors. *Cancer Res.,* **48**, 3630–3

60. Mivechi, N. F. and Li, G. C. (1985). Thermotolerance and profile of protein synthesis in murine bone marrow cells after heat shock. *Cancer Res.,* **45**, 3843–9

61. Mivechi, N. F. and Li, G. C. (1990). Heat sensitivity, thermotolerance and protein synthesis of granulocyte and macrophage progenitors from mice and from long-term bone marrow cultures. *Int. J. Hyperthermia,* **6**, 529–41

62. Dunn, F. and Fry, F. J. (1971). Ultrasonic threshold dosages for the mammalian central nervous system. *I.E.E.E. Trans. Bio-Med. Eng.,* **18**, 253–6

63. Fry, F. J., Ades, W. J. and Fry, W. J. (1958). Production of reversible changes in the central nervous system by ultrasound. *Science,* **127**, 83–4

64. Fry, F. J., Kossoff, G., Eggleton, R. C. and Dunn, F. (1970). Threshold ultrasonic dosages for structural changes in the mammalian brain. *J. Acoust. Soc. Am.,* **6**, 1413–17

65. Stuhlfauth, K. (1952). Neural effects of ultrasonic waves. *Br. J. Phys. Med.,* **15**, 10–14

66. Takagi, S. F., Higashino, S., Shibuya, T. and Osawa, N. (1959). The actions of ultrasound on the myelinated nerve, the spinal cord and the brain. *Jap. J. Physiol.,* **10**, 183–93

67. Young, R. R. and Henneman, E. (1961). Reversible blockage of nerve conduction by ultrasound. *Arch. Neurol.,* **4**, 83–9

68. Necker, R. (1988). Central thermosensitivity: CNS and extra-CNS. In Hales, J. R. S. (ed.) *Thermal Physiology,* pp. 53–61. (New York: Raven Press)

69. van der Knaap, M. S., Valk, J., Bakker, C. J., Schooneveld, M., Faber, J. A. J., Willemse, J. and Gooskens, R. H. J. M. (1991). Myelination as an expression of the functional maturity of the brain. *Dev. Med. Child Neurol.,* **33**, 849–57

70. Davison, A. N. and Dobbing, J. (1966). Myelination as a vulnerable period in brain development. *Br. Med. Bull.,* **22**, 40–4

71. Rodier, P. M. (1980). Chronology of neuron development: animal studies and their clinical implications. *Dev. Med. Child Neurol.,* **22**, 525–45

72. Rakic, P. (1977). Prenatal development of the visual system in rhesus monkey. *Phil. Trans. R. Soc. London,* **278**, 245–60

73. Howard, E. (1973). DNA content of rodent brains during maturation and aging and autoradiography of postnatal DNA synthesis in monkey brain. *Progr. Brain Res.,* **40**, 91–114

74. Raaf, J. and Kernohan, J. W. (1994). A study of the external granular layer in the cerebellum: the disappearance of the external granular layer and the growth of the molecular and internal granular layer in the cerebellum. *Am. J. Anat.,* **75**, 151–72

75. Rakic, P. and Sidman, R. L. (1970). Histogenesis of cortical layers in human cerebellum, particularly the lamina dissecans. *J. Comp. Neurol.,* **139**, 473–500

76. Ellisman, M. H., Palmer, D. E. and Andre, M. P. (1987). Diagnostic levels of ultrasound may disrupt myelination. *Exp. Neurol.,* **98**, 78–92

77. Siddiqi, T. A., Meyer, R. A., Woods, J. R. and Plessinger, M. A. (1988). Ultrasound effects on fetal auditory brain stem responses. *Obstet. Gynecol.,* **72**, 752–6

78. Duggan, P. M., Liggins, G. C. and Barnett, S. B. (1993). Pulsed ultrasound and electrocortical activity in fetal sheep. *Early Hum. Dev.,* **35**, 121–7

79. Rao, G. S., Abraham, V., Fink, B. A., Margulies, N. and Ziskin, M. C. (1989). Biochemical changes in the developing central nervous system due to hyperthermia. *Teratology,* **41**, 327–32

80. Margulies, N., Abraham, V., Way, J. S. and Ziskin, M. C. (1993). Reversible biochemical changes in the developing rat central nervous system following ultrasound exposure. *Ultrasound Med. Biol.,* **17**, 383–90

81. Suneetha, N. and Surendra Kumar, R. P. S. (1993). Ultrasound-induced enhancement of ACH, ACHE and GABA in fetal brain tissue of mouse. *Ultrasound Med. Biol.,* **19**, 411–13

82. Holland, C. K., Deng, C. X., Apfel, R. E., Alderman, J. L., Fernandez, L. A. and Taylor, K. J. W. (1996). Direct evidence of cavitation *in vivo* from diagnostic ultrasound. *Ultrasound Med. Biol.*, **22**, 917–25

83. Tarantal, A. F. and Canfield, D. R. (1994). Ultrasound-induced lung hemorrhage in the monkey. *Ultrasound Med. Biol.*, **20**, 65–72

84. Dalecki, D., Child, S. Z., Raeman, C. H., Penney, D. P., Mayer, R., Cox, C. and Carstensen, E.L. (1997). Thresholds for fetal haemorrhages produced by a piezoelectric lithotripter. *Ultrasound Med. Biol.*, **23**, 287–97

85. Parent, R. A. (1992). *Treatise on Pulmonary Toxicology*, vol. I. *Comparative Biology of the Normal Lung.* (Boca Raton: CRC Press)

86. AIUM/NEMA (1992). Output Display Standard (ODS). *Standard for Real-Time Display of Thermal and Mechanical Acoustic Indices on Diagnostic Ultrasound Equipment.* (Bethesda, MD: American Institute of Ultrasound in Medicine)

Sensitivity to diagnostic ultrasound in obstetrics

6

S. B. Barnett

SUMMARY

Embryonic and fetal tissues are sensitive to damage by physical agents and the consequences of exposure depend on the stage of development and tissue composition. These factors also influence the ultrasound exposure at the tissue target. The sensitivity of mammalian tissue is related to its functional status, and actively dividing tissues in the embryo and fetus are susceptible to damage. Should the interaction with ultrasound be sufficient to cause cell death, mitotic delay, or defects in cell growth during organogenesis, the effects would manifest as physical deformities which would be readily detectable. However, if a small volume of tissue in the focal zone of the ultrasound beam is perturbed it is possible that the consequences may not be detected unless the target tissue is a critical sensory pathway or organ. Reports of increased incidence of left-handedness and delayed speech development in children exposed to ultrasound *in utero* have been suggested as evidence of ultrasound interference with the process of neural cell migration in the second and third trimesters.

Radiation pressure can cause the displacement and streaming of fluid, e.g. of cerebrospinal fluid in brain ventricles, or of oocytes in follicles, but there is no evidence of adverse health risk associated with diagnostic procedures. The likelihood of inertial cavitation occurring increases if the biological medium is a liquid containing gas bubbles. Hence, the introduction of echo-contrast agents into biological media can increase their sensitivity to interaction with ultrasound. The presence of a tissue/gas boundary provides an interface for non-thermal interactions. Insonating laboratory animals with maximum output from diagnostic equipment results in capillary bleeding in the lungs. There is no evidence of such cavitation-related damage in fetal lungs, which are not inflated.

Ultrasound-induced heating is greatest in tissue containing bone, and biologically significant temperature increases can be expected in the fetus from the second trimester, if the beam is kept stationary for more than 30 s in pulsed Doppler applications. Some sensory organs are encased in bone and may be susceptible to heating by conduction, e.g. the pituitary and neuroepithelium of the inner ear. Organs with poor circulation, such as the optic lens, are susceptible to significant heating by ultrasound.

There have been some reports in animals and humans of retarded growth and development following frequent exposures to diagnostic ultrasound in the absence of significant heating. These effects are difficult to explain from current knowledge on ultrasound mechanisms. More research is needed for full understanding of the possible biological mechanisms involving growth factors. Reports of fetal responses and transient electrophysiological responses show that ultrasound can be detected by the central nervous system (CNS). However, this does not necessarily imply that the bioeffect is hazardous to the fetus.

INTRODUCTION

The consequence of exposure of biological tissue to diagnostic ultrasound can be quite variable and depends on the susceptibility of the cells to damage and on their functional status.

To draw conclusions on the susceptibility of certain tissues to ultrasound presupposes that all conceivable mechanisms of interaction are fully understood and quantifiable. Research has made progress in some areas and the mechanisms that have received most attention are those of thermal and cavitational origin. Interest in bioeffects and safety of ultrasound in medicine has increased in recent years. The World Federation for Ultrasound in Medicine and Biology (WFUMB) has taken a leading role by sponsoring international symposia to evaluate the status of research into thermal[1] and non-thermal[2] mechanisms. The sensitivity of various biological tissues to damage by ultrasound has not yet been specifically addressed.

The purpose of this chapter is to identify structures that are sensitive to the effects of ultrasound and to present information as it relates to interpretation of risk from exposure to diagnostic ultrasound. It is intended to complement other chapters in this book that describe the biological effects of diagnostic ultrasound.

Developing embryonic and fetal tissues are sensitive to exposure to various physical agents, including ultrasonic energy. The result of an interaction with ultrasound depends on the stage of development, the tissue composition and its functional status. At preimplantation (1–2 weeks after fertilization), adverse physical stress often results in abortion of the developing embryo. During postimplantation, the early development of the central nervous system, the cardiovascular system and other organ systems occurs. Should cell death, mitotic delay, or defects in cell growth occur during this stage of organogenesis, the effects would manifest as physical deformities in the fetus. At 5–10 weeks of pregnancy (after the last menstrual period), trauma will result in neural tube defects. Development of the human forebrain proceeds by neuroblast division from 10 to 20 weeks of pregnancy. The capacity for repair and compensation of neural deficits progressively decreases during fetogenesis. Loss of neurons, caused by ultrasound exposure, would have little chance of replacement by unplanned neuroblast division and the deficiency could result in maldevelopment and impairment of mental function. If a small volume of tissue in the focal zone of the ultrasound beam is perturbed, it is possible that the consequences may not be detected unless the target tissue is a critical sensory pathway or organ such as the eye or ear, or a relatively large proportion of the body volume, e.g. the early embryo.

The upper surface of the posterior portion of the cerebral temporal lobe in the human brain is responsible for the development of speech and is predominantly controlled by the left hemisphere[3]. This region develops at around the 31st week of pregnancy, whereas the right side develops at approximately 29 weeks. The human brain is asymmetric and the dominance by the left hemisphere creates a high incidence of right-handedness in the community. The concept of cerebral dominance is well known in clinical neurology. If the cerebral cortex on one side of the fetal brain is damaged, or cell division is significantly delayed, the cortical region of the other hemisphere will take over and allow the change to left-handedness.

As all cortical neurons are generated by mitotic cell division in the neural tube, an important process in fetal brain development is the migration of these neural cells from the subcortical zone into the cortex and the formation of neural synapses. Cellular migration to the cortex is completed between 6 and 8 months of pregnancy. Perturbation of this process can produce subtle neurophysiological effects.

NON-THERMAL SENSITIVITY

The likelihood that ultrasound exposure may cause damage to the embryo or fetus depends on the acoustic conditions and on whether or not the insonated biological tissue can sustain the physical mechanisms of interaction. The different composition of various biological tissues attributes differing susceptibility to the effects of diagnostic ultrasound. Fluid substances allow the occurrence of certain non-thermal mechanisms which might result in biological effects. Those associated with bulk fluid streaming caused by radiation pressure are described in Chapter 9.

Cavitation is a non-thermal mechanism of interaction that involves the formation, oscillation and occasional collapse of bubbles in a sound field. The subject is comprehensively described in a book by Leighton[4]. A precondition for inertial (previously termed transient or collapse) cavitation is the existence of gas bodies, i.e. gaseous inclusions. At high-peak negative pressures inertial cavitation can cause cavities or bubbles in liquids to collapse and release energy sufficiently intense to disrupt molecular bonds and produce chemically reactive free radicals[5]. These free radicals may interfere with DNA, causing chromosomal damage. Although this has been reported in cell studies, it has not been directly observed in patients or in laboratory animals exposed to diagnostic intensities.

There is no substantiated evidence that exposure to diagnostic ultrasound is capable of directly altering chromosomes, or that subthreshold doses accumulate to produce a delayed effect. Although some studies have reported an increase in the rate of sister chromatid exchange in mammalian cells following exposure to diagnostic ultrasound, the weight of evidence indicates that the effect is more likely to be due to a secondary condition of the experiment rather than being directly attributable to ultrasound interaction[6,7].

Cell culture studies allow exposed cells to grow in liquid media isolated from the effect of surrounding tissue, thereby minimizing bulk heating and increasing the likelihood of cavitation. The endpoints studied are usually gross effects on cell survival or mutagenicity. Cells normally grow at a regulated rate in a systematic pattern in response to contact stimuli. When this contact inhibition is lost, cell growth becomes haphazard, leading to tumor formation. Normal growth relies on feedback from the cell membrane. The plasma membrane of the cell is sensitive to its environment and signals changes inwardly, to the cell nucleus, and outwardly, by communicating with its neighbors, e.g. by synaptic transmission. There is growing evidence that responses to quite weak environmental changes are amplified through a signal transduction pathway that can ultimately alter gene expression and critical cell functions. The outer surface of the bilayer lipid plasma membrane is composed of a matrix of carbohydrate chains that form the glycocalyx. Electrochemical gradients exist across cell membranes and alterations can influence the passage of ions into or out of the cell. For example, the intracellular calcium concentration controls protein synthesis. It has been suggested that changes brought about by the action of low-intensity therapeutic pulsed ultrasound[8] involve altered membrane permeability and enhanced release of growth factors from mast cells in response to the relatively low-level effects of stable cavitation. Molecular vibration of cell surface receptors is thought to mediate the influx of calcium ions.

Detection of cell membrane effects requires sophisticated biochemical techniques that have rarely been applied to studies of the biological effects of ultrasound. There are insufficient data currently available to assess risk at the subcellular level, where the most sensitive structure may be the cell membrane and the signal transduction pathway. Free radicals are readily produced within cells during the process of amplification of surface (i.e. cell membrane) responses to the cells' external environment. These reactive chemical species usually have a very short life unless it is extended by other environmental factors. Free radicals can also be formed in the extracellular fluid as a result of inertial cavitation. It is generally assumed that the time needed to penetrate the cell plasma membrane and to reach the nucleus is longer than the survival time of these chemical species.

The presence of a tissue/gas boundary provides an interface for cavitation-related interactions resulting in damage in the mammalian lung at low-level exposures with pulsed ultrasound[9]. This bioeffect has since been consistently repeated in different animal species and has been verified in different laboratories[10,11]. As the onset of cavitation can occur within a diagnostic pulse, these bioeffects have been observed after exposures as brief as 20 s[12]. From published data on acoustic output measurements (see Chapter 3) it is evident that the peak rarefaction pressure threshold for lung hemorrhage in small animals is achievable at the maximum outputs of some modern ultrasonographic equipment operating Doppler systems. No such effect is observed in soft tissue of the liver, in the absence of gas bodies, unless the pulse intensity is increased to therapeutic levels. There is no evidence of lung tissue damage in the fetus, in which the lungs are not filled with air.

Other non-thermal effects include ultrasound-induced streaming. Modern diagnostic ultrasound equipment produces sufficient radiation pressure to cause bulk movement of fluids along the ultrasound propagation path. It is possible that the forces exerted on the developing embryo or fetus might disrupt cell organization or neural cell migration. The health implications of radiation pressure and streaming were considered in a recent symposium on safety of ultrasound in medicine[2]. In a discussion of this subject in Chapter 9, radiation stress is recognized as a potential bioeffect mechanism that should be considered in first-trimester ultrasound examinations.

Evidence that mild exposure to ultrasound can elicit a significant biological response is seen in the growing number of publications on the therapeutic benefit of ultrasound interaction with tissue. Pulsed ultrasound was shown to enhance the rate of tissue growth and repair in varicose ulcers[8]. More recently, accelerated rates of bone growth and fracture repair have been reported following insonation with low-intensity outputs ($30 \, mW/cm^2$, $1.5 \, MHz$) in rats[13] and humans[14]. The FDA has recently approved for therapeutic use in the USA an ultrasound instrument (Sonic Accelerated Fracture Healing System, Exogen, Inc.). Although the piezoelectric nature of bone material has been recognized for some time, the biological processes by which bone growth is enhanced at these low levels of acoustic power is not fully understood. The fact that there is evidence of tissue reaction to low-level ultrasound exposure raises some interesting questions about the possible stimulatory effects of ultrasound on fetal bone growth centers. The brief duration of exposure in normal imaging procedures suggests that a significant effect may be unlikely. Information on threshold exposures for the therapeutic effect only applies to non-fetal situations.

There have been reports of increased incidence of non-right-handedness[15] and delayed speech development[16] in children who were exposed to diagnostic ultrasound while in the uterus. Impedance of migration of fetal neural cells is known to result in such conditions[3] and this effect has been suggested as evidence of ultrasound-induced interference in fetal brain development. The findings of impaired speech development were not supported in a different epidemiology study[17]. This research requires substantiation by independent duplication. There is a higher incidence of left-handedness and associated learning disorders in males, in the general population. This aspect of sex-related effects should be considered in epidemiology studies on possible associations with ultrasound exposure.

Fetal responses

There have been reports of increased fetal activity during ultrasound examinations, and the question of a possible fetal response has not been thoroughly explored. Findings of studies on fetal activity in humans exposed to continuous wave ultrasound emitted by fetal heart rate monitors are conflicting. In studies in which the mother evaluated fetal movement, increased fetal activity was reported in one[18] and no change was found in others[19,20]. Animal studies have been undertaken to determine whether exposure to diagnostic ultrasound can be detected by a fetal neural response. Transient changes in the auditory brainstem response have been reported in near-term fetal sheep exposed to pulsed ultrasound from a clinical diagnostic scanner[21]. A study using chronically instrumented fetal sheep[22] found no change in the electro-corticogram during exposure to low-intensity pulsed ultrasound. In this study the fetal lamb was not anesthetized and the ultrasound transducer was remotely energized by computer control during the normal behavioral and physiological state.

The phenomenon of 'microwave hearing' is a common effect of human exposure to electromagnetic radiation. The mechanism of action is considered to be thermoelastic expansion in the neural tissue of the brain. The key feature is the rapid rate of temperature rise[23], whereas the magnitude of temperature increase is negligible, being considerably less than 0.1 °C. A similar 'audible' response effect was recently reported by patients during transcranial Doppler examinations of the basilar artery[24]. The mechanism has yet to be explained. It is possible that a similar effect is detected in fetal exposures. These transient responses to a physical stimulus should not, necessarily, be taken as a biologically significant event.

The suggestion of a non-specific stress response in the developing fetus exposed to diagnostic ultrasound is offered in reports of reduced birth weight in monkeys[25] and in humans[26].

THERMAL SENSITIVITY

All physiological processes in mammalian biological systems are controlled and affected by temperature. The rate of metabolism, enzyme reactions and protein synthesis is directly affected by temperature. Changes from the normal physiological temperature can have important consequences for sensitive tissues. The protein structure of cell membranes is subject to alteration by changes in temperature. The subject of bioeffects resulting from ultrasound-induced heating is described in detail in Chapter 4.

The temperature increase that may be produced in mammalian tissue during an ultrasonic examination depends on the properties of both the ultrasound field parameters (described in Chapters 2 and 3) and the biological tissue. In this context, the important properties of biological tissue are the acoustic absorption coefficient, thermal conduction and blood perfusion. The tissue absorption characteristics determine how much heat is deposited. Body fluids (e.g. amniotic fluid, cerebrospinal fluid, urine) have low acoustic absorption, approximately 0.003 dB/cm per MHz) and, therefore, have little risk of unwanted ultrasound-induced temperature increase. However, ultrasound propagation through a path of low-attenuating fluid (e.g. an

obstetric acoustic window through the urine-filled maternal bladder) can allow finite amplitude distortion of the wave. The increased energy content of the travelling wave is deposited at an absorbing interface, resulting in substantially greater heating than would be expected for a normal sinusoidal wave[1,27]. On the other hand, if the propagation path is through soft tissue, then the amount of energy reaching the target is reduced by an amount according to the attenuating properties of the tissue.

The absorption coefficient of mammalian biological tissue increases with increasing protein content and is particularly high in collagen[28,29]. The average value for brain tissue is 0.2 dB/cm per MHz. The highest value (10 dB/cm per MHz) occurs in mineralized bone, giving it the greatest potential for undesirable ultrasound-induced temperature increase. The final tissue temperature depends on thermal conduction into neighboring tissues and blood perfusion dissipating heat. In organs such as the liver, kidney and brain, the perfusion rate is permanently high, so that the heat dissipation is effective. However, in fatty tissue, periosteum and bone, the perfusion rate is low, so that these tissues are susceptible to heating by ultrasound.

Mineralization and ossification of bone begins in the 12th week of pregnancy. The amount of ultrasound-induced heating correlates with gestational age and bone development; fetal bone structures become increasingly prone to heating with advancing pregnancy. Thermal insult to the embryo can produce bioeffects that are readily detectable since they are likely to be amplified during fetal development. However, the likelihood of producing a significant temperature increase in soft embryonic tissue is lower than in the bony tissue of the fetus. In late pregnancy, the ultrasound beam is small relative to the size of the fetus, so that tissue damage and associated bioeffects may be difficult to detect.

Although the tissues of the CNS have a low absorption coefficient, they are encased in the bone of the fetal skull and vertebrae which is readily heated by ultrasound. For example, the adjacent soft tissue of the cerebral cortex and the pituitary will be heated by conduction. The neurons of the developing fetal brain are susceptible to ultrasound-induced heating[1]. A temperature increase of around 4.5 °C has been measured in the brain in late-gestation live guinea-pig fetuses after exposure for 2 min to pulsed ultrasound *in utero*. The pulsing conditions are similar to those available for pulsed Doppler applications[30,31] (described in detail in Chapter 4).

Sensory organs would be expected to be sensitive to ultrasound-induced mechanical stimulation or heating. A study in mammals examined the sensitivity of the retina to exposure to low-intensity B-mode pulsed ultrasound for extended duration and found no microscopically detectable changes in the neural epithelium[32]. Because the lens of the eye is composed of highly absorbing collagen fibers and has no blood supply, it is susceptible to ultrasound-induced heating. In its original regulatory policy for premarket approval of ultrasonographic imaging devices, the FDA limited the output intensity of ultrasonographic equipment according to the intended application[33]. That involving ophthalmic examination was allocated the strictest limit, being one-fifth of the level allowed for fetal examinations. The effects of clinical exposures from modern diagnostic exposures to pulsed Doppler ultrasound have not been adequately addressed.

While having low absorption properties themselves, sensory structures are often located close to bone. For example, the inner ear is surrounded by the dense petrous bone and its neuroepithelium is readily destroyed by therapeutic exposures to continuous wave ultrasound[34]. The potential for ultrasound-induced heating causing damage to small, important structures lying close to bone, such as the developing pituitary or hypothalamus, has not been fully studied. However, adverse effects on cell division have been reported in bone marrow following exposure to pulsed ultrasound similar to maximum pulsed Doppler outputs[35]. It is unlikely that exposure to scanned-mode ultrasonographic imaging will produce significant heating in embryonic or fetal tissue[1].

There is an extensive database showing hyperthermia to be teratogenic in many animal species[36]. Data are derived from whole-body heating of pregnant animals. Ultrasound-induced heating of the CNS causes relatively small volumes of tissue (equivalent to the focal zone of the ultrasound beam) to be heated rapidly. For example, a 3 °C temperature increase can occur within 30-s exposure at fetal bone/soft tissue interfaces[31]. This is approximately 1/60th of the time required to elevate the core temperature by the same amount using whole-body incubation. The volume of tissue heated by ultrasound is restricted to that enveloped by the ultrasound beam, that lying close to the transducer (e.g. in intracavitory applications), or that adjacent to strongly absorbing tissue such as bone. There are few scientific data on the direct teratogenic effects that might result from small volumes of localized tissue heating caused by an ultrasound beam.

There is some evidence to suggest that ultrasound-induced bioeffects can be potentiated by modest increases in temperature[1,37,38]. There may be an increased risk for febrile patients from hyperthermic damage[1], since their elevated core temperature would add to the ultrasound-induced heating of the embryo or fetus. In general, the embryo or fetus is considered to be particularly susceptible to the effects of ultrasound-induced heating.

The World Federation for Ultrasound in Medicine and Biology has published recommendations[1] that represent international consensus on safety of ultrasound in medicine. The recommendations are duplicated here, as they are relevant in the context of sensitivity to ultrasound of embryonic and fetal tissues compared with adult biological tissues.

WFUMB recommendations (1992)

(1) Based solely on a thermal criterion, a diagnostic exposure that produces a maximum temperature rise of 1.5 °C above normal physiological levels (37 °C) may be used without reservation in clinical examinations.

(2) The possible influence of potentiating factors should be considered. This indicates

that Doppler ultrasound in a febrile patient might present an additional embryonic and fetal risk.

(3) Exposure of adult proliferative tissues to heat can cause damage comparable to that occurring in the embryo and fetus, but with exposures to 42 °C for up to 2 h complete recovery is expected.

CLINICAL SIGNIFICANCE

The clinical relevance of any tissue lesion depends on the physiological function that is disturbed, the severity of damage and the possibility of compensation or repair. The brain cannot replace lost functional cells, but small sites of damage would not be detected unless they involved sensory organs (eye, inner ear), nerve conduction, or CNS function. Small localized lesions of parenchymatic organs (kidney, liver, thyroid, etc.) can be repaired and are of little consequence. Propagation of any form of energy in biological systems has the potential to elicit a reaction. The results of such an interaction may, or may not, be biologically significant. It is important to understand the distinction between bioeffects and biohazards when potential risk to human health is considered.

In embryonic structures, any lesion carries the risk of abnormal further development with the consequence of malformation of various organs or body parts. The type, localization and clinical relevance of a defect depends more on the stage of embryological development than on the type of insult. Moderate temperature increases which are capable of arresting cell proliferation might be of no consequence in adult tissue, but can derange the normal embryonic development and thus induce neural tube defects such as anencephaly or spina bifida, or produce congenital heart malformations or cleft lip and palate.

Within the fetal hematopoietic system, the bone marrow is the main site of blood formation in the third trimester of pregnancy. Different types of biological effects have been observed following exposure to pulsed ultrasound. One study used the bone marrow in femurs of adult guinea pigs as a model for fetal brain development[35] where actively dividing cells are close to bone. The exposure simulated pulsed Doppler output in a fixed ultrasound beam of sufficient intensity to maintain a temperature increase of 2.5 °C above normal body temperature. Cell division was disturbed, resulting in the production of abnormal nuclei in neutrophils after exposure for 6 min. It is possible to produce a similar temperature increase in the fetal brain with pulsed Doppler (see Chapter 4), but it is unlikely that the beam could be held stationary for long enough to cause the observed degree of abnormal cell division. Other studies of effects at modest temperature increase[39] have reported significantly reduced production of neutrophils and monocytes[40] and growth-related effects[25,41] in monkey fetuses following frequent exposure to diagnostic ultrasound throughout pregnancy. The sensitivity of the hematopoietic system to diagnostic ultrasound exposure is described in Chapter 5.

While there have been some reports of effects on the chromosomes following *in vitro* insonation under specialized laboratory conditions that favor the existence of inertial cavitation, mutation events from *in vivo* exposures are much less likely. Structural chromosome aberrations and point mutations mostly have adverse clinical consequences, while the biological significance of an altered rate of sister chromatid exchange is obscure. Dividing cells are more sensitive to mutagenic effects than non-dividing cells. Therefore, embryonic and fetal tissues may be assumed to have a higher sensitivity to mutagenic agents. There is at present no indication that medical ultrasound is capable of inducing mutations in mammalian tissue *in vivo*.

In vitro studies with mammalian cells have demonstrated mutagenic effects under conditions of severe acoustic shock where the production of inertial (collapse) cavitation was associated with the production of ultraviolet light, a known mutagen. These findings cannot be directly extrapolated to *in vivo* effects in mammalian tissue. A conclusion reached by the recent international *WFUMB Symposium on the Safety of Ultrasound in Medicine*[2] was that while *in vitro* studies provide a useful insight into the non-thermal mechanisms by which ultrasound can produce biological effects, 'caution is required in applying these results to medical ultrasound exposures *in vivo*'.

Generally, the types of experimental bio-effect studies that have been carried out have tested for rather gross endpoints. Effects such as fetal weight reduction represent a systematic breakdown of the developmental processes of the developing organism. Potentially more important are interruptions in development in localized anatomical regions, particularly in neural tissue. These effects would not be detected by studies that evaluated gross morphology, or even cytology. The kinetics of intracellular biochemical processes are clearly temperature-sensitive but research has been limited on the potential ultrasound effects on such endpoints.

Lung hemorrhage has been reported at diagnostic exposures in postnatal life, but there has been no report of a cavitation-induced bioeffect in the fetus, to date. The lungs of the fetus do not contain gas to enable cavitationally-induced bioeffect in obstetric examinations. However, the potential risk cannot be excluded that ultrasound exposure may cause lung hemorrhage, particularly in a premature neonate, by an inappropriately conducted cardiographic examination performed at maximum pulsed Doppler output.

Body fluids saturated with gas molecules and protein nuclei might provide sites for bubble formation and cavitation. The likelihood of inertial cavitation occurring increases if the biological medium is a liquid containing gas bubbles. The use of echo-contrast materials to enhance sonographic imaging may increase the sensitivity of mammalian tissue to ultrasound interaction and provide opportunities for cavitation. Hence, the introduction of echo-contrast agents into biological media can increase its sensitivity to interaction with ultrasound.

With the establishment of changes in the regulatory process leading toward self-regulation, there is a potential for higher tissue exposures from the increasing use of complex sophisticated ultrasonographic equipment in wider applications. Meanwhile, there is a growing trend towards using ultrasound in obstetrics at earlier stages of embryonic development in the first trimester. This led the European Committee for Ultrasound Radiation Safety to publish cautionary notes on the routine use of pulsed Doppler in early pregnancy[42,43].

There have been some reports in humans and animals of retarded growth and development following frequent exposures to diagnostic ultrasound (see Chapters 5 and 10), in the absence of significant heating. These effects are difficult to explain from current knowledge on ultrasound mechanisms.

A paper by members of the WFUMB Safety Committee recently examined the issue of sensitivity of biological tissue to medical ultrasound[44]. It recognized the absence of scientific data and advised that little work has been undertaken specifically to assess the sensitivity of various kinds of biological tissues to damage by ultrasound. The paper also commented that, even if small volumes of tissue, equivalent to the focal zone of an ultrasound beam, were affected, it is possible that the consequences would not be detected unless a critical sensory structure was involved.

Reports of fetal responses and transient electrophysiological responses show that ultrasound can be detected by the CNS. However, this does not necessarily imply that the bioeffect is hazardous to the fetus.

References

1. Barnett, S. B. and Kossoff, G. (eds.) (1992). Issues and recommendations regarding thermal mechanisms for biological effects of ultrasound. In World Federation for Ultrasound in Medicine and Biology Symposium on Safety and Standardisation in Medical Ultrasound. *Ultrasound Med. Biol.*, **18**, Special issue, No.9

2. Barnett, S. B. (ed.) (1997). Conclusions and recommendations on thermal and non-thermal mechanisms for biological effects of ultrasound. In World Federation for Ultrasound in Medicine and Biology Symposium on Safety of Ultrasound in Medicine. *Ultrasound Med. Biol.*, in press

3. Geschwind, N. and Galaburda, A. M. (1985). Cerebral lateralization. Biological mechanisms, associations, and pathology: 1. A hypothesis and a program for research. *Arch. Neurol.*, **42**, 428–59

4. Leighton, T. G. (1994). *The Acoustic Bubble.* (London: Academic Press)

5. NCRP (1983). *Biological Effects of Ultrasound: Mechanisms and Clinical Implications*, Report 74. (Bethesda, MD: National Council on Radiation Protection and Measurements)

6. Barnett, S. B. (1990). *Investigation into the biological effects of pulsed ultrasound with emphasis on potential mutagenicity.* PhD Thesis, University of N.S.W. School of Medicine, Sydney, Australia

7. Barnett, S. B. (1996). Ultrasound safety in obstetrics: what are the concerns? *Ultrasound Q.*, **13**, 228–39

8. Dyson, M. (1991). The susceptibility of tissues to ultrasound. In Docker, M. F. and Duck, F. A. (eds.) *The Safe Use of Diagnostic Ultrasound*, pp. 24–29. (London: British Institute of Radiology)

9. Child, S. Z., Hartman, C. L., Schery, L. A. and Carstensen, E. L. (1990). Lung damage from exposure to pulsed ultrasound. *Ultrasound Med. Biol.*, **16**, 817–25

10. Tarantal, A. F. and Canfield, D. R. (1994). Ultrasound induced lung haemorrhage in the monkey. *Ultrasound Med. Biol.*, **20**, 65–72

11. Holland, C. K., Deng, C. X., Apfel, R. E., Alderman, J. L., Fernandez, L. A. and Taylor, K. J. W. (1996). Direct evidence of cavitation *in vivo* from diagnostic ultrasound. *Ultrasound Med. Biol.*, **22**, 917–25

12. Raeman, C. H., Child, S. Z., Dalecki, D., Cox, C. and Carstensen, E. L. (1996). Exposure time dependence of the threshold for ultrasonically induced murine lung haemorrhage. *Ultrasound Med. Biol.*, **22**, 139–41

13. Wang, S., Lewallen, D. G., Bolander, M. E., Chao, E. Y. S., Ilstrup, D. M. and Greenleaf, J. F. (1994). Low intensity ultrasound treatment increases strength in a rat femoral fracture model. *J. Orthop. Res.*, **12**, 40–7

14. Heckman, S. D., Ryaby, J. P., McCabe, J., Frey, J. J. and Kilcoyne, R. F. (1994). Acceleration of tibial fracture healing by non-invasive, low-intensity pulsed ultrasound. *J. Bone Joint Surg.*, **76A**, 26–34

15. Salvesen, K. A., Vatten, L. J., Eik-Nes, S. H., Hugdahl, K. and Bakketeig, L. S. (1993). Routine ultrasonography *in utero* and subsequent handedness and neurological development. *Br. Med. J.*, **307**, 159–64

16. Campbell, J. D., Elford, R. W. and Brant, R. F. (1993). Case–control study of prenatal ultrasonography exposure in children with delayed speech. *Can. Med. Assoc. J.*, **149**, 1435–40

17. Salvesen, K. A., Vatten, L. J., Bakketeig, L. S. and Eik-Nes, S. H. (1994). Routine ultrasonography *in utero* and speech development. *Ultrasound Obstet. Gynecol.*, **4**, 101–3

18. David, H., Weaver, J. B. and Pearson, J. F. (1975). Doppler ultrasound and fetal activity. *Br. Med. J.*, **2**, 62–4.

19. Murrills, A. J., Barrington, P., Harris, P. D. and Wheeler, T. (1983). Influence of Doppler ultrasound on fetal activity. *Br. Med. J.*, **286**, 1009–12.

20. Hertz, R. H., Timor-Tritsch, I., Dierker, L. J. and Rosen, M. (1979). Continuous ultrasound and fetal movement. *Am. J. Obstet. Gynecol.*, **135**, 152–4

21. Siddiqi, T. A., Meyer, R. A., Woods, J. R. and Plessinger, M. A. (1988). Ultrasound effects on fetal auditory brain stem responses. *Obstet. Gynecol.*, **72**, 752–6

22. Duggan, P. M., Liggins, G. C. and Barnett, S. B. (1993). Pulsed ultrasound and electrocortical activity in fetal sheep. *Early Hum. Dev.*, **35**, 121–7

23. Saunders, R. D., Kowalczuk, C. I. and Sienkiewicz, Z. J. (eds.) (1991). *Biological Effects of Exposure to Non-Ionising Electromagnetic Fields and Radiation: III Radiofrequency and microwave radiation*, NRPB-R240. (Chilton, Didcot, UK: National Radiological Protection Board)

24. Magee, T. R. and Davies, A. H. (1993). Auditory phenomena during transcranial Doppler insonation of the basilar artery. *J. Ultrasound Med.*, **12**, 747–50

25. Tarantal, A. F. and Hendrickx, A. G. (1989). Evaluation of the bioeffects of prenatal ultrasound exposure in the cynomolgus macaque (*Macaca fascicularis*): 1. Neonatal/infant observations. *Teratology*, **39**, 137–47

26. Newnham, J. P., Evans, S. F., Michael, C. A., Stanley, F. J. and Landau, L. I. (1993). Effects of frequent ultrasound during pregnancy: a randomised controlled trial. *Lancet*, **2**, 887–91

27. Bacon, D. R. and Carstensen, E. L. (1990). Increased heating by diagnostic ultrasound due to nonlinear propagation. *J. Acoust. Soc. Am.*, **88**, 26–34.

28. Duck, F. A. (1990). *Physical Properties of Tissue: A Comprehensive Reference Book.* (London: Academic Press)

29. NCRP (1992). *Exposure Criteria for Medical Diagnostic Ultrasound: 1. Criteria Based on Thermal Mechanisms*, Report no. 113. (Bethesda, MD: National Council for Radiation Protection and Measurements)

30. Horder, M. M., Barnett, S. B., Edwards, M. J. and Kossoff, G. (1993). *In vivo* temperature rise in the fetus from duplex Doppler ultrasound. In *Proceedings of the 23rd Annual Scientific Conference of the Australian Society of Ultrasound in Medicine*, Melbourne, Australia, September

31. Horder, M. M., Barnett, S. B., Edwards, M. J. and Kossoff, G. (1997). *In utero* measurement of ultrasound-induced heating in guinea-pig fetal brain, abstr. 2300. In *Proceedings of the 41st Annual Convention of AIUM*, p.22, San Diego, USA, March

32. Barnett, S. B. and Kossoff, G. (1977). Negative effects of long duration pulsed ultrasound on the retina of cats. In White, D. and Brown, R. E. (eds.) *Ultrasound in Medicine Engineering Aspects*, vol. 3, pp. 2025–32. (New York and London: Plenum Press)

33. FDA (1985). *510(k) Guide for Measuring and Reporting Acoustic Output of Diagnostic Ultrasound.* (Rockville, MD: Food and Drug Administration, Center for Devices and Radiological Health). (1992 updated Draft document)

34. Barnett, S. B. (1980). The effect of ultrasonic irradiation on the structural integrity of the inner ear labyrinth. *Acta Otolaryngol.*, **89**, 424–32

35. Barnett, S. B., Edwards, M. J. and Martin, P. (1991). Pulsed ultrasound induces temperature elevation and nuclear abnormalities in bone marrow cells of guinea pig femurs. In *6th World Congress of Ultrasound in Medicine*, abstr. 3405. (Denmark: WFUMB)

36. Edwards, M. J. (1993). Hyperthermia and birth defects. *Cornell Vet.*, **83**, 1–7

37. Angles, J. M., Walsh, D. A., Li, K., Barnett, S. B. and Edwards, M. J. (1990). Effects of pulsed ultrasound and temperature on the development of rat embryos in culture. *Teratology*, **42**, 285–93

38. Barnett, S. B., Walsh, D. A. and Angles, J. A. (1990). Novel approach to evaluate the interaction of pulsed ultrasound with embryonic development. *Ultrasonics*, **28**, 166–70

39. Tarantal, A. F., Chu, F., O'Brien, W. D. and Hendrickx, A. G. (1993). Sonographic heat generation *in vivo* in the gravid long-tailed macaque (*Macaca fascicularis*). *J. Ultrasound Med.*, **5**, 285–95

40. Tarantal, A. F., Gargosky, S. E., Ellis, D. S., O'Brien, W. D. and Hendrickx, A. G. (1995). Hematologic and growth-related effects of frequent prenatal ultrasound exposure in the long-tailed macaque (*Macaca fascicularis*). *Ultrasound Med. Biol.*, **21**, 1073–81

41. Tarantal, A. F. and Hendrickx, A. G. (1993). Evaluation of the bioeffects of prenatal ultrasound exposure in the cynomolgus macaque (*Macaca fascicularis*): 3. Developmental and haematological studies. *Teratology*, **47**, 159–70

42. EFSUMB (1995). European Committee for Ultrasound Radiation Safety – the Watchdogs, Clinical Safety Statement, 1994. *Eur. J. Ultrasound*, **2**, 77

43. EFSUMB (1996). European Committee for Ultrasound Radiation Safety – The Watchdogs, Clinical Safety Statement, 1995. *Eur. J. Ultrasound*, **3**, 283

44. Barnett, S. B., Rott, H. D., Ter Haar, G. R., Ziskin, M. C. and Maeda, K. (1997). The sensitivity of biological tissue to ultrasound. *Ultrasound Med. Biol.*, **23**, 805–12

Cavitation produced by diagnostic ultrasound pulses: can it occur *in vivo?*

7

C. K. Holland

SUMMARY

Current ultrasound diagnostic systems can produce cavitation *in vitro* and *in vivo.* Experimental evidence of cavitation-related bioeffects is seen as capillary bleeding in animal tissues. Several animal models have exhibited a threshold for petechial hemorrhage in lung within the current output of diagnostic ultrasound systems, but the implications for human exposure are not yet determined. The World Federation for Ultrasound in Medicine and Biology has concluded that acoustic cavitation can alter mammalian tissue and that it is important to consider its significance in medical applications of ultrasound. In the absence of gas bodies, or pre-existing pockets of gas, the threshold for damage is much higher. This last point is significant, because most ultrasound examinations in obstetrics and gynecology are performed predominantly in tissues with no identifiable gas bodies. For this reason, the fetus is not considered to be at risk of lung damage from acoustic cavitation. A mechanical index has been developed to gauge the potential for cavitation. The introduction of echo-contrast media substantially lowers the exposure threshold required to produce cavitation.

INTRODUCTION

Ultrasound has provided an enormous wealth of knowledge in diagnostic medicine, particularly in obstetrics. It is estimated that millions of ultrasound examinations are performed each year and ultrasound remains one of the fastest growing imaging modalities. This growth is due to many factors including its low cost, real-time information, and, to no lesser extent, its apparent lack of bioeffects. Despite the large number of ultrasound examinations performed to date, there are very few indications that clinical applications of diagnostic ultrasound have caused harmful biological effects on the patient or operator.

The use of diagnostic ultrasound to monitor fetal development and to assess disease continues to increase because of improvements in resolution and the expansion of clinical applications of Doppler modes for the evaluation of blood flow. Increased resolution and flow discrimination have been accomplished, in part, by the utilization of higher acoustic frequencies and thus higher acoustic output levels due to increased attenuation (see Chapter 3). Concern for potential bioeffects at these levels has prompted concerted action by the Food and Drug Administration (FDA), American Institute of Ultrasound in Medicine (AIUM) and National Electrical Manufacturers Association (NEMA) to draft an acoustical output display standard for diagnostic ultrasound equipment[1]. In addition, the World Federation of Ultrasound in Medicine and Biology (WFUMB) has sponsored a series of symposia which have resulted in internationally agreed recommendations on the safe use of ultrasound in medicine following examination of potential biological effects and the clinical safety of diagnostic ultrasound[2].

For the first time clinicians are being presented with real-time data on acoustic output of diagnostic scanners and are being asked not only to understand the manner in which ultrasound propagates through and interacts with tissue, but also to gauge the potential for adverse bioeffects.

INERTIAL CAVITATION

What is it?

Cavitation refers to the formation and dynamic behavior of gas bubbles. The term 'cavitation' was first coined in 1895 by Thornycroft and Barnaby in the hydrodynamic context of the observation of separation of water from a ship's propeller in motion[3]. Acoustic cavitation is the growth of bubbles from microscopic pockets of undissolved gas and/or vapor, stabilized on solid surfaces or by surface-active films, due to the reduction in pressure in the negative phase of the acoustic cycle.

The inception of acoustic cavitation is demarcated by a specific threshold value: the minimum acoustic pressure necessary to initiate the growth of a cavity in a fluid during the rarefaction phase of the cycle. A number of parameters affect this threshold, including: initial bubble or 'nucleus' size, acoustic pulse characteristics (such as center frequency, pulse repetition frequency and pulse duration), ambient hydrostatic pressure and host fluid properties (such as density, viscosity, compressibility, heat conductivity and surface tension). Inertial, formerly called 'transient', cavitation is the growth of short-lived bubbles which undergo large variations from their equilibrium sizes during pressure changes in a few acoustic cycles. During contraction, the surrounding fluid inertia controls the bubble motion[4]. Large acoustic pressures are necessary to generate inertial cavitation, and the collapse of these cavities is often violent.

Prediction of inertial cavitation from diagnostic ultrasound

Flynn developed a comprehensive mathematical formalism for theoretically investigating the dynamics of spherical cavitation bubbles that are damped by heat conduction within the cavity, and viscosity and compressibility of the surrounding fluid[4,5]. The formulation consisted of non-linear ordinary differential equations which were solved numerically. Maximum collapse pressures and temperatures within the cavity and collapse speeds of the cavity were presented for a range of nucleus sizes.

Apfel derived an approximate expression that predicted the conditions under which inertial cavitation would occur[6] and determined that acoustic cavitation was a possible consequence of diagnostic ultrasound[7]. He concluded that although ultrasonic heating effects were a function of energy dose, the presence or absence of cavitation nuclei and the time history of the insonifying pressure wave were more appropriate parameters when discussing the potential for cavitation. This approximate theory was extended by Holland and Apfel to include the effects of surface tension, viscosity and inertia in the treatment of bubble motion[8]. Their results yielded information about the cavitation threshold behavior at a given frequency over a range of initial nucleus sizes.

Flynn also utilized the equations he previously developed to provide the quantitative physical basis for the generation of inertial cavitation by microsecond pulses of ultrasound such as those used clinically for diagnostic purposes[9]. Flynn assumed that the effects of diffusion, evaporation and condensation may be ignored and that the amount of gas originally in the nucleus remains constant throughout the motion. Even more importantly, it was assumed that the cavity retains its spherical shape even though the interface of a real collapsing cavity is dynamically unstable and may break up. Shown in Figure 1 are plots of the 2.25 MHz frequency insonifying tone-burst utilized for the calculations and the normalized curve of radius vs. time. The peak pressure amplitude was 0.5 MPa, with a pulse duration of 1 μs. The initial nucleus radius, R_n, was 1 μm. As seen from the plot, the bubble grows over the three acoustic cycles to four times its original size, collapses rapidly and rebounds.

The gas content of a cavity plays a minor role in the bubble's dynamics until its collapse, which is rapidly decelerated by the trapped gas.

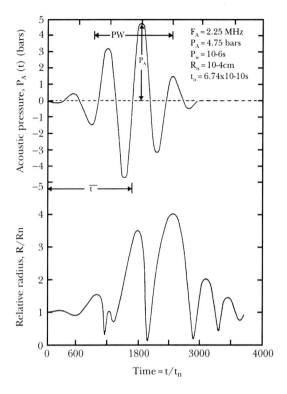

Figure 1 Insonifying pressure pulse (top) and resulting cavity motion (bottom). Reprinted from Flynn 1982 with permission from AIP

The collapse can be so rapid that the motion is adiabatic, causing the pressure and temperature in the interior of the cavity to rise by hundreds of megapascals and thousands of degrees Kelvin, respectively. These temperatures are momentarily high enough to cause −OH free radical formation[10], which might damage surrounding biological material in much the same way that ionizing radiation does. Free radical formation has been demonstrated experimentally by Suslick and co-workers[11] in alkane solutions of metal carbonyls through the use of comparative rate thermometry. One consequence of such free radical formation is the generation of a light flash, a phenomenon known as sonoluminescence[12,13].

High-pressure shock waves that emanate from collapsing bubbles can mechanically damage surrounding material. Inertial cavitation is, therefore, an effective mechanism for concentrating energy. It transforms the relatively low energy density of the ultrasonic field into a high-energy density characteristic of the neighborhood of a collapsing bubble. Both mechanical disruption and free radical production are consequences of inertial cavitation and present a cause for concern in some diagnostic ultrasound applications. It is important to search for regions where cavitation could occur *in vivo* along with the possible biological manifestations of damage.

Pre-existing cavitation nuclei may be one of the principal controlling factors in mechanical interactions which lead to biological effects. The body is such an excellent filter that nucleation sites may be found in only small numbers and only at selected sites. For instance, if water is passed through a filter with a 2-μm pore diameter, the cavitation threshold pressure doubles. The theoretical tensile strength of water which is completely devoid of any heterogeneity is about 100 MPa. Various models have been suggested to explain bubble formation in animals[14,15] and these models have been used extensively in cavitation threshold determination. One model[16] is used in the prediction of scuba diving tables and as such also has applicability to the patient *in vivo*. It remains to be seen how well such models will predict the nucleation of bubbles in the body from diagnostic ultrasound.

EVIDENCE OF CAVITATION *IN VIVO*

It is possible to generate bubbles *in vivo* from the short-duration, high-amplitude acoustic pulses used by extracorporeal shock wave lithotripters (ESWL). The peak positive, or compressional pressure (p_c) for lithotripsy pulses can be as much as 50 MPa and the negative, rarefactional pressure (p_r) around 20 MPa. Finite amplitude distortion causes high frequencies to appear in high-amplitude ultrasound fields. Although ESWL pulses have significant energy at high frequencies due to finite amplitude distortion, a large portion of the energy is actually in the 100-kHz frequency range, much lower than that of diagnostic ultrasound scanners. The lower frequency makes cavitation more likely. There is evidence to indicate that the destruction of gall stones or renal calculi may be due to the effects of collapsing bubbles[17-19]. As evidence of the destructive power, when cavitation due to application of extracorporeal shock wave lithotripsy occurs next to a solid surface, a high-velocity liquid jet may form during collapse, generating a sufficient impulse to produce observable damage on metal surfaces[20]. If one takes a sheet of aluminum foil and places it at the focus of a lithotripter, small pinholes will be generated[21]. The impact is even sufficient to pit solid brass and aluminium plates.

Lithotripsy and diagnostic ultrasound differ in the acoustic power generated and are not comparable in the bioeffects produced. Some diagnostic devices produce peak rarefactional pressures greater than 3 MPa, which is in the lower range of lithotripter outputs[22-24]. Interestingly, lung damage and surface petechiae have been noted as side-effects of ESWL in clinical cases[25]. Inertial cavitation (described above) was suspected as the cause of this damage and has prompted several researchers to study the effects of diagnostic ultrasound exposure on lung parenchyma.

Hemorrhage in lung and intestine

Lung tissue has proven to be an important tissue to determine the bioeffects from diagnostic ultrasound. The presence of air in the alveolar spaces constitutes a significant source of gas bodies. Child and colleagues[26] measured pressure thresholds for hemorrhage in mouse lung exposed to 1–4 MHz short-pulse diagnostic ultrasound (i.e. 1–10 μs pulse durations). The threshold of damage in murine lung at these frequencies was established to be 1.4 MPa, which is below the current maximum allowed limit of output of clinical ultrasound scanners. Pathological features of this tissue damage included extravasation of blood cells into the alveolar spaces[27]. Their findings suggest that the damage evoked by ultrasound affects the microvasculature, or capillary-size vessels, only. It was hypothesized that cavitation, originating from gas-filled alveoli, was responsible for the damage. Their data are the first to provide direct evidence that clinically relevant, pulsed ultrasound exposures produce deleterious effects in mammalian tissue in the absence of significant heating. Hemorrhagic foci induced by 4-MHz pulsed Doppler have also been reported in the monkey[28]. Damage in the monkey lung was of a significantly lesser degree than that in the mouse. Subsequently, thresholds for lung damage from pulsed diagnostic ultrasound have been assessed in the neonatal mouse[29], neonatal pig[30], rat[31], rabbit and pig[32,33]. Ultrasonically induced petechial hemorrhage has also been observed in the mouse intestine[34,35]. In all of these animal systems, pockets of gas have been activated during ultrasonic exposure. In these studies, it was impossible to show categorically that these effects were induced by bubbles, because the cavitation-induced bubbles were not observed. Further studies are required to determine the relevance of these findings to the human.

The gross organization and cellular composition of the lung is similar in mammals, although there are significant physiological and anatomical differences related to the organization of the distal airways, alveolar morphology and blood supply[36]. Morphological studies have demonstrated that capillaries within the alveolar septa of most mammals are arranged as a single layer separated from the air spaces by a thin cellular barrier (100 nm). Owing to this anatomical configuration, Tarantal and Canfield[37] hypothesized that these regions are more susceptible to conditions where bubble oscillation and rupture may occur. They also noted that an important factor specific to the lung may be the monolayer of surfactant within the alveoli. Surfactant, the alveolar lining fluid, is responsible for modifying surface tension in order to promote lung expansion and prevent lung collapse. It is possible that, during exposure to ultrasound, microbubbles are created within edges of the surfactant-rich alveolus. These microbubbles may oscillate and collapse, causing localized disruption of the epithelial/endothelial barrier and subsequent extravasation of red blood cells into the alveolar space. Holland and Apfel have previously shown a direct correlation between a reduction in the cavitation threshold and reduced host fluid surface tension[38,39].

Present results indicate that current diagnostic scanners are capable of producing inertial cavitation *in vivo*. As an example of the potential relevance of this work, premature infants often present with cardiopulmonary problems requiring echocardiography to monitor heart development and pathology. In these infants, unlike the fetus *in utero,* alveoli are filled with air. This respiratory gas may form nuclei for acoustic cavitation within the parenchyma. In addition, these infants often exhibit cardiopulmonary compromise and are given surfactant therapy to aid in the exchange of gases in the alveoli. The volume of already compromised lung, the presence of surfactant, and the frequency of ultrasound scans of premature infants are cause for careful consideration by the practitioner and for further research. Lung surfactant therapy administered in premature infants with respiratory distress syndrome could potentially exacerbate cavitation-mediated damage in lungs if exposed to high levels of ultrasound. Therefore, the effect of such exogenous surfactants on ultrasound-induced lung damage should be explored.

Although it is a proven phenomenon *in vitro*[40], the occurrence of cavitation *in vivo* due to diagnostic ultrasound has been difficult to document in mammalian systems, primarily because of the transient nature of its occurrence (i.e. microseconds) and the localized character of the resultant effects (i.e. < 10 μm). In order to explore the hypothesis of cavitation-based bioeffects from diagnostic ultrasound, Holland and colleagues[31] determined the thresholds of damage in rat lungs exposed to 4.0-MHz pulsed Doppler and color Doppler ultrasound. In this study, a 30-MHz frequency acoustic detection scheme[41] was used to provide the first direct evidence of cavitation from diagnostic ultrasound pulses. Damage was observed with histological features consistent with those seen in mice and monkeys due to diagnostic ultrasound exposures. However, in this limited study, bubble activity was not correlated with histological damage. The question remains: do bubbles, if produced by diagnostic ultrasound *in vivo,* cause significant biological effects?

POTENTIAL FOR CAVITATION *IN VIVO*

Use of ultrasound echo-contrast agents in obstetrics and gynecology

Transvaginal sonography can detect gross Fallopian tubal disease[42] and is routinely used for follicular monitoring[43] and oocyte retrieval[45,46] in the infertility clinic setting. It is current practice to administer exogenous ultrasound echo-contrast agents, or microbubbles, to visualize Fallopian tubal patency[46]. In addition, sonohysterography is currently employed as a technique for endometrial evaluation and involves the instillation of sterile saline under continuous sonographic visualization to assess the endometrial cavity[47]. The saline undoubtedly contains many microbubbles which, like the bubble-based echo-contrast agents themselves, could potentially serve as cavitation nuclei (see Chapter 8). Although no significant adverse physiological reactions have occurred with this use of contrast agents, it would seem prudent to improve our understanding of the interaction of ultrasound with such agents.

Indicator of risk of cavitation

Recent proposals concerning the regulation of acoustic output from medical ultrasound systems have suggested greatly increasing the role that the physician and/or sonographer will play in limiting the potential for ultrasound bioeffects. Informed decision concerning the possible adverse effects of ultrasound in comparison to desired diagnostic information will probably become more important over the next few years. In this regard, information would be provided to the operator concerning the relative potential for bioeffects but would allow the physician the discretion to increase the acoustic output beyond a level which might induce a biological response. To assist in the decision concerning the potential for producing adverse non-thermal effects, given the range of different imaging conditions utilized clinically, a mechanical index was developed as part of a Real-Time Output Display Standard which gives the operator an indication of the proximity to a cavitational threshold[1].

The mechanical index, or MI, was developed by Apfel and Holland[48]. Theoretical calculations for cavitation prediction have yielded a rough trade-off between peak rarefactional pressure and frequency. This predicted trade-off assumes short-pulse (a few acoustic cycles) and low-duty cycle ultrasound ($< 1.0\%$). This relatively simple result can be used to gauge the potential for the onset of cavitation from diagnostic ultrasound. The mechanical index is defined as:

$$MI = \frac{P}{\sqrt{f}}$$

where P is the peak negative pressure in the acoustic field which is derated according to 0.3 dB/cm per MHz to allow for *in vivo* attenuation and is normalized by 1 MPa, and f is the center frequency of the transducer. The derated pressure represents an estimation of the peak rarefactional pressure *in situ*. The MI was adopted by the FDA, AIUM and NEMA as a real-time output display to estimate the potential for cavitation-related adverse bioeffects *in vivo*. As indicated before, the collapse temperatures for inertial cavitation are very high. For this index, a collapse temperature of 5000 K was chosen on the basis of the potential for free radical generation. The frequency dependence of the pressure required to generate this thermal threshold takes a relatively simple form. The MI is a 'mechanical energy index' because the square of the MI is roughly proportional to mechanical work that can be performed on a bubble in the acoustic rarefaction phase. Inherent in the formulation of the MI are the conditions only for the 'onset' of inertial cavitation. The degree to which the threshold is exceeded, however, does relate to the degree of bubble activity that may occur, and the amount of bubble activity may correlate with the probability of an undesirable bioeffect. Note that, given our present knowledge, exceeding the cavitation threshold does not mean that there will be a bioeffect caused by inertial cavitation. Below an MI of 0.7, the physical conditions probably do not exist to promote bubble growth even in the presence of a broad size distribution of bubble nuclei in the body.

As the MI is intended to predict the likelihood of non-thermal bioeffects, it will need to address the issues relating to hemorrhage in the lung and intestine tissue/gas interfaces where the mechanism is not yet fully understood. Studies which explore the occurrence and degree of damage above threshold values are essential for the knowledge base which will guide practitioners on the interpretation and use of the MI as a real-time display standard.

Safety guidelines

Several official positions concerning the status of bioeffects from ultrasound should be considered. Both the AIUM and the WFUMB publish updated conclusions and recommendations for ultrasound bioeffects[1,2,49]. The most important item to note is the high level of confidence in clinical safety statements (see WFUMB statement on clinical safety, below). However, due to recent data exhibiting hemorrhage in animal lung and intestine exposed to clinical diagnostic levels of ultrasound (described above), the WFUMB is more cautious (see WFUMB statement on tissue/gas interfaces, below).

WFUMB conclusion on clinical safety (1997)

No adverse effects on patients or instrument operators caused by exposure at acoustic output levels typical of currently available, properly operating diagnostic ultrasound instruments have ever been established. Current data indicate that the benefits to patients of the prudent use of diagnostic ultrasound outweigh the risks, if any, that may be present.

WFUMB conclusion on tissue/gas interfaces (1997)

Tissue/gas interfaces are known to exist in the postnatal lung and intestinal lumina. These interfaces greatly increase the potential for non-thermal biological effects. Evidence from mammalian studies shows that pulmonary capillary bleeding can occur at diagnostic ultrasonic pressure levels. Within the frequency range of present diagnostic instruments (2–10 MHz), the threshold for pulmonary capillary bleeding is approximately 1 MPa and the threshold for intestinal bleeding is approximately 3 MPa. Ultrasonically induced lung damage in the fluid-filled lungs of fetuses is not to be expected.

CONTROL OF THE ACOUSTIC OUTPUT POWER

Perhaps the most important aspect of a discussion of potential bioeffects is how the physician or sonographer can minimize these effects. Without some ability to control the acoustic output of the ultrasound system, knowledge of potential bioeffects has limited utility. Several specific methods can be used to limit ultrasound exposure while maintaining diagnostically relevant images. The foremost of these is to use a low output power. The output power control might be labelled 'intensity', 'output' or 'transmit' on a clinical ultrasound system. The receiver gain rather than the output power should be increased to minimize the amount of exposure. In the context of minimizing the potential for cavitation, an output with a low MI (< 1) should be used and the use of unscanned modes (Doppler and M-mode) should be avoided where there may be tissue/gas interfaces present. The selection of the appropriate transducer will also limit the need for high acoustic power.

At present, the USA Food and Drug Administration regulates the maximum output of ultrasound systems produced in the USA to an established level through a marketing approval process that requires the output of devices to be equivalent to those produced prior to 1976. This historic regulation has provided a safety margin for ultrasound while allowing clinically useful performance. Because it might be diagnostically advantageous to increase the output limit (e.g. patients with large amounts of subcutaneous fat are difficult to scan), ultrasound systems might produce higher outputs in the near future. Recent proposals regarding the regulation of acoustic output of medical ultrasound systems have suggested greatly increasing the role of the physician and/or sonographer in limiting the potential for ultrasound bioeffects. Patients also need to be reassured about the safety of a diagnostic ultrasound scan. There is no substitute for a well instructed operator. Real-time display of the mechanical index on diagnostic scanners will help clinicians evaluate and minimize potential risks in the use of such instrumentation.

References

1. American Institute of Ultrasound in Medicine. (1992). *Standard for Real-time Display of Thermal and Mechanical Acoustic Indices on Diagnostic Ultrasound Equipment.* (Laurel, MD: AIUM)
2. Barnett, S. B. (ed.) (1997). Conclusions and recommendations on thermal and non-thermal mechanisms for biological effects of ultrasound. *World Federation for Ultrasound in Medicine and Biology Symposium on Safety of Ultrasound In Medicine. Ultrasound Med. Biol.*, in press
3. Thornycroft, J. and Barnaby, S. W. (1895). *Inst. Civ. Eng.*, **122**, 51
4. Flynn, H. G. (1975). Cavitation dynamics, I. A mathematical formulation. *J. Acoust. Soc. Am.*, **57**, 1379–96
5. Flynn, H. G. (1975). Cavitation dynamics. II. Free pulsations and models for cavitation bubbles. *J. Acoust. Soc. Am.*, **58**, 1160–70
6. Apfel, R. E. (1982). Acoustic cavitation: a possible consequence of biomedical uses of ultrasound. *Br. J. Cancer*, **45**, 140–6
7. Apfel, R. E. (1986). Possibility of microcavitation from diagnostic ultrasound. *IEEE Trans. UFFC*, **32**, 139–42
8. Holland, C. K. and Apfel, R. E. (1989). An improved theory for the prediction of microcavitation thresholds. *IEEE Trans. UFFC*, **36**, 204–8
9. Flynn, H. G. (1982). Generation of transient cavities in liquids by microsecond pulses of ultrasound. *J. Acoust. Soc. Am.*, **72**, 1926–32
10. Carmichael, A. J., Mossaba, M. M., Riesz, P. and Christman, C. L. (1986). Free radical production in aqueous solutions exposed to simulated ultrasonic diagnostic conditions. *IEEE Trans. UFFC*, **32**, 148–55

11. Suslick, K. S., Hammerton, D. A. and Cline, R. E. Jr (1986). The sonochemical hot spot. *J. Am. Chem. Soc.*, **108**, 5641–2

12. Verrall, R. E. and Seghal, C. M. (1988). Sonoluminescence. In Suslick, K. S. (ed.) *Ultrasound: Its Chemical, Physical and Biological Effects*, pp. 227–86. (New York: VCH)

13. Crum, L. A. and Fowlkes, J. B. (1986). Acoustic cavitation generated by microsecond pulses of ultrasound. *Nature (London)*, **319**, 52–4

14. Harvey, E. N., Barnes, D. K., McElroy, W. D., Whiteley, A. H., Pease, D. C. and Cooper, K. W. (1944). Bubble formation in animals, I. Physical factors. *J. Cell. Compar. Phys.*, **24**, 1–22

15. Harvey, E. N., Barnes, D. K., McElroy, W. D., Whiteley, A. H., Pease, D. C. and Cooper, K. W. (1944). Bubble formation in animals. II. Gas nuclei and their distribution in blood and tissues. *J. Cell. Compar. Phys.*, **24**, 23–34

16. Yount, D. E. (1978). Skins of varying permeability: a stabilization mechanism for gas cavitation nuclei. *J. Acoust. Soc. Am.*, **65**, 1429–39

17. Coleman, A. J., Saunders, J. E., Crum, L. A. and Dyson, M. (1987). Acoustic cavitation generated by an extracorporeal shockwave lithotripter. *Ultrasound Med. Biol.*, **15**, 213–27

18. Delius, M., Brendel, W. and Heine, G. (1988). A mechanism of gallstone destruction by extracorporeal shock wave. *Naturwissenschaften*, **75**, 200–1

19. Williams, A. R., Delius, M., Miller, D. L. and Schwarze, W. (1989). Investigation of cavitation in flowing media by lithotripter shock waves both *in vitro* and *in vivo*. *Ultrasound Med. Biol.*, **15**, 53–60

20. Crum, L. A. (1988). Cavitation microjets as a contributory mechanism for renal calculi disintegration in ESWL. *J. Urol.*, **140**, 1587

21. Coleman, A. J., Saunders, J. E., Crum, L. A. and Dyson, M. (1987). Acoustic cavitation generated by an extracorporeal shockwave lithotripter. *Ultrasound Med. Biol.*, **13**, 69–76

22. Patton, C. A., Harris, G. R. and Phillips, R. A. (1994). Output levels and bioeffects indices from diagnostic ultrasound exposure data reported to the FDA. *IEEE Trans. UFFC*, **41**, 353–9

23. Duck, F. A., Starritt, H. C., Aindow, J. D. and Hawkins, A. J. (1985). The output of pulse-echo ultrasound equipment: a survey of powers, pressures and intensities. *Br. J. Radiol.*, **58**, 989–1001

24. Duck, F. A., Starritt, H. C. and Anderson, S. P. (1987). A survey of the acoustic output of ultrasonic Doppler equipment. *Clin. Phys. Physiol. Meas.*, **8**, 39–49

25. Chaussy, C., Schmiedt, E., Jocham, D., Fuchs, G., Brendel, W., Forssmann, B. and Hepp, W. (1986). *Extracorporeal Shock Wave Lithotripsy*. (Basel: Karger)

26. Child, S. Z., Hartmen, C. L., Schery, L. A. and Carstensen, E. L. (1990). Lung damage from exposure to pulsed ultrasound. *Ultrasound Med. Biol.*, **16**, 817–25

27. Penney, D. P., Schenk, E. A., Maltby, K., Hartman-Raeman, C., Child, S. Z. and Carstensen, E. L. (1993). Morphological effects of pulsed ultrasound in the lung. *Ultrasound Med. Biol.*, **19**, 127–35

28. Tarantal, A. F. and Canfield, D. R. (1994). Ultrasound-induced lung hemorrhage in the monkey. *Ultrasound Med. Biol.*, **20**, 65–72

29. Frizzell, L. A., Chen, E. and Chong, L. (1994). Effects of pulsed ultrasound on the mouse neonate: hind limb paralysis and lung hemorrhage. *Ultrasound Med. Biol.*, **20**, 53–63

30. Baggs, R., Penney, D. P., Cox, C., Child, S. Z., Raeman, C. H., Dalecki, D. and Carstensen, E. L. (1996). Thresholds for ultrasonically induced lung hemorrhage in neonatal swine. *Ultrasound Med. Biol.*, **22**, 119–28

31. Holland, C. K., Zheng, X., Apfel, R. E., Alderman, J. L., Fernandez, L. and Taylor, K. J. W. (1996). Direct evidence of cavitation *in vivo* from diagnostic ultrasound. *Ultrasound Med. Biol.*, **22**, 917–25

32. Zacchary, J. G. and O'Brien, W. D. (1995). Lung lesions induced by continuous- and pulsed-wave (diagnostic) ultrasound in mice, rabbits and pigs. *Vet. Pathol.*, **32**, 43–54

33. Dalecki, D., Child, S. Z., Raeman, C. H., Cox, C. and Carstensen, E. L. (1997). Ultrasonically-induced lung haemorrhage in young swine. *Ultrasound Med. Biol.*, **23**, 777–81

34. Miller, D. L. and Thomas, R. M. (1995). Thresholds for hemorrhages in mouse skin and intestine induced by lithotripter shock waves. *Ultrasound Med. Biol.*, **21**, 249–57

35. Dalecki, D., Raeman, C. H., Child, S. Z. and Carstensen, E. L. (1995). Intestinal haemorrhage from exposure to pulsed ultrasound. *Ultrasound Med. Biol.*, **21**, 1067–72

36. Tyler, W. S. and Julian, W. D. (1992). Gross and subgross anatomy of lungs, pleura, connective tissue septa, distal airways, and structural units. In Parent, R. A. (ed.) *Treatise on Pulmonary Toxicology*, vol. I. *Comparative Biology of the Normal Lung*, pp. 35–58. (Boca Raton, FL: CRC Press)

37. Tarantal, A. F. and Canfield, D. R. (1994). Ultrasound-induced lung haemorrhage in the monkey. *Ultrasound Med. Biol.*, **20**, 65–72

38. Holland, C. K. and Apfel, R. E. (1989). An improved theory for the prediction of microcavitation thresholds. *IEEE Trans. UFFC*, **36**, 204–8

39. Holland, C. K. and Apfel, R. E. (1990). Thresholds for transient cavitation produced by

pulsed ultrasound in a controlled nuclei environment. *J. Acoust. Soc. Am.*, **88**, 2059–69

40. Holland, C. K., Roy, R. A., Apfel, R. E. and Crum, L. A. (1992). *In vitro* detection of cavitation induced by a diagnostic ultrasound system. *IEEE Trans. UFFC.*, **39**, 95–101

41. Roy, R. A., Madanshetty, S. and Apfel, R. E. (1990). An acoustic backscattering technique for the detection of transient cavitation produced by microsecond pulses of ultrasound. *J. Acoust. Soc. Am.*, **87**, 2451–55

42. Timor-Tritsch, I. E. and Rottem, S. (1987). Transvaginal ultrasonographic study of the fallopian tube. *Obstet. Gynecol.*, **70**, 331–4

43. Drugan, A., Blumenfeld, Z., Erlik, Y., Timor-Tritsch, I. E. and Brandes, J. M. (1989). The use of transvaginal sonography in infertility. In Timor-Tritsch, I. E. and Rottem, S. (eds.) *Transvaginal Sonography,* pp. 143–59. (London: Heineman Medical Books)

44. Feichtinger, W. and Demeter, P. (1984). Laparoscopic or ultrasonically guided follicle aspiration for *in vitro* fertilization. *J. In Vitro Fertil. Embryo Transfer,* **1**, 244–9

45. Daya, S., Wikland, M., Nilsson, L. and Enk, L. (1987). Fertilization and embryo development of oocytes obtained transvaginally under ultrasound guidance. *J. In Vitro Fertil. Embryo Transfer,* **4**, 338–42

46. Volpi, E., Zuccaro, G., Patriarca, A., Rustichelli, S. and Sismondi, P. (1996). Transvaginal sonographic tubal patency testing using air and saline solution as contrast media in a routine infertility clinic setting. *Ultrasound Obstet. Gynecol.,* **7**, 43–8

47. Cullinan, J. A., Fleischer, A. C., Kepple, D. M. and Arnold, A. L. (1995). Sonohysterography: a technique for endometrial evaluation. *RadioGraphics,* **15**, 501–14

48. Apfel, R. E. and Holland, C. K. (1991). Gauging the likelihood of cavitation from short-pulse, low-duty cycle diagnostic ultrasound. *Ultrasound Med. Biol.,* **17**, 179–85

49. American Institute of Ultrasound in Medicine (1993). *Bioeffects and Safety of Diagnostic Ultrasound.* (Laurel, MD: AIUM)

Echo-contrast agents: what are the risks?

8

J. B. Fowlkes and E. Y. Hwang

SUMMARY

Echo-contrast agents are being examined for specific obstetric and gynecological applications such as Fallopian tube patency assessment, although currently their principal use is vascular assessment through signal enhancement of blood flow in organs such as the kidney and liver and in the myocardium. Animal studies have shown that the presence of these gas bodies reduces the acoustic pressure amplitude required to induce cavitation-related bioeffects, such as hemolysis. A recommendation of the World Federation for Ultrasound in Medicine and Biology safety symposium (1996) on echo-contrast agents is that, 'gas bodies introduced by a contrast agent increase the probability of cavitation'. The potential of echo-contrast agents to enhance cavitational effects in obstetric examinations has not been thoroughly investigated. In addition, the agents are affected by diagnostic ultrasound fields, as shown by the reduction in signal enhancement and production of stimulated acoustic emissions during ultrasound imaging. There have been few reported adverse effects from clinical studies using such agents, and these were primarily associated with sensations at the time of injection.

INTRODUCTION

This chapter provides an overview of echo-contrast agents and their application together with an assessment of potential bioeffects and safety considerations in obstetrics and gynecology. Echo-contrast agents are a relatively new addition to ultrasound technology, but are being researched at an accelerating rate because of their high potential based on observations during experimental trials and the impact contrast agents have made on other imaging modalities such as X-ray computed tomography and magnetic resonance imaging. Similar or better success is anticipated for ultrasound contrast agents, and therefore more companies are developing agents that are now in various stages of preclinical and clinical trials, with some agents already available for selected clinical applications.

HISTORY OF ULTRASOUND CONTRAST AGENTS

Gramiak and colleagues[1] first reported increased echogenicity in M-mode cardiac images following the injection of indocyanine. The source of the contrast was later attributed to air-filled microbubbles produced by the rapid injection of the solution through a small-bore needle[2,3]. A pressure drop in the fluid at the needle tip causes gas bubbles to form through a process known as hydrodynamic cavitation. The term acoustic cavitation refers to the pulsation of gas bubbles in an acoustic field (see Chapter 7). Hydrodynamic cavitation is the formation and response of bubbles due to pressure changes in the liquid which result from fluid flow (hydrodynamics). A good example of its existence and effects is the fact that ship propellers can generate significant underwater noise and are eroded prematurely due to hydrodynamic cavitation. When the bubbles were formed by Gramiak and colleagues[1], the increased scattering of ultrasound by gas, orders of magnitude greater than by a particle such as a red blood cell of the same size, provided the added contrast observed. There are a number of excellent reviews on ultrasound contrast agents[4-12]. In one of the reviews[4], agents were classified into five types: free gas bubbles, encapsulated gas bubbles, colloidal suspensions, emulsions and aqueous solutions.

This overview describes gas bubble contrast agents which have the highest potential for ultrasound-induced bioeffects and represent the largest number of agents under development. Most contrast agents use gas bubbles in a solution that can be injected into the bloodstream. The principal difficulty with free bubble contrast agents, such as those noted by Gramiak and co-workers, is the lack of persistence after injection into a gas-saturated solution such as human blood. The increased internal gas pressure in the bubble due to surface tension at the liquid/gas interface causes the gas to diffuse into the solution, and the bubble rapidly dissolves. However, acoustic cavitation thresholds in water are unusually low, indicating that gas pockets in the liquid are somehow stabilized. Several models have been proposed to explain the cavitation results, including crevices in hydrophobic particles[13,14] and skins or shells surrounding the bubble which prevent diffusion[15]. Such a stabilization mechanism is important to those interested in developing ultrasound contrast agents based on gas bubbles.

One of the first encapsulated microbubbles used a gelatin shell enveloping nitrogen gas[16]. However, these bubbles were quite large (mean diameter of 80 μm) and their applications were restricted, owing to lung filtration. In 1984, Rasor Associates developed the first transpulmonary agent – a particle which trapped small pockets of gas. However, despite its early success, this was not fully developed, owing to complications over production and clinical approval.

In the investigation of sonicated solutions for microbubble contrast agents, it was discovered that a sonicated solution of 5% albumin produced stable bubbles of a size range which were particularly effective in transpulmonary applications[17]. The mean diameter was approximately 4 μm with 95% of the bubble less than 10 mm in diameter and a concentration of 10^8 bubbles/ml. This agent was commercialized as Albunex®

(Molecular Biosystems Inc., San Diego, CA) and was the first to obtain the approval of the Food and Drug Administration (FDA) in the USA, in 1994. Its current clinical application is in echocardiography, but it is also being investigated for urinary reflux and Fallopian tube patency.

Meanwhile, Schering AG (Berlin) developed a saccharide-based gas bubble contrast agent by mixing special microparticles with a galactose solution immediately before injection. Their first product, SH U 454 or Echovist®, was registered in Germany in 1991. The bubbles have a mean diameter of 3 μm but their lack of stability has limited usage to right heart applications[18]. As was the case for Albunex, this product has also been used in obstetric and gynecological applications (summarized later). Schering's more recent product, SH U 508A or Levovist®, is a different formulation that is mixed with sterile water and is significantly more robust. Contrast enhancement from this agent can be observed in locations beyond the heart such as the kidneys, liver and brain.

Within the last few years there has been a large increase in the number of companies that have developed agents that are at various stages of clinical and preclinical evaluation.

Lipid-encapsulated bubble contrast agents have been investigated by a number of groups. The agent Filmix® (CavCon Inc., Farmington, CT) is reported to increase the echogenicity in some tumors including rat brain and liver[19]. It is administered intravenously but its low bubble concentration does not provide contrast enhancement as a vascular agent. The agent Aerosomes® (ImaRx Pharmaceuticals, Tucson, AZ) and its next generation formulation MRX115®, demonstrates contrast enhancement beyond the heart following intravenous administration[20,21].

UltraVue® (Delta Biotechnology Limited, Nottingham, UK) is composed of gas-filled albumin spheres which are resuspended in water as a colloidal suspension prior to injection. The spheres measure 3–10 μm in diameter and the albumin shell has a thickness of 100–200 nm. Measurements made by de Jong and co-workers[22] indicate that the sphere is quite rigid and provides no resonance effects (see explanation below) in the diagnostic frequency range for attenuation or scattering of ultrasound.

The Bubbicles® agent was developed from the earlier iodipamide ethyl ester (IDE) solid particle agent[23]. The new Bubbicle particles have rough surfaces, which allow them to trap gas and significantly improve echogenicity. The particles are collected in the Kupffer cells of the liver and provide a negative contrast for cancer lesions having a poorly developed reticulo-endothelial system. The Kupffer cells can each collect as many as 30 particles and enhance liver parenchyma detail for up to 120 min.

A new agent from Sonus Inc. (EchoGen®) is an emulsion of stabilized perfluorocarbon particles at room temperature. The perfluorocarbon (dodecafluoropentane) has a boiling point of around 30 °C and, therefore, becomes a gas after injection into the body. The low solubility of the gas and its low diffusivity provide Doppler enhancement for several minutes[24].

Numerous other agents are under development and many could be classed as second-generation agents such as FS069® (Molecular Biosystems Inc.). Many of these agents such as FS069®, MRX-115® and AF0150® (Imagent US, Alliance Pharmaceuticals) use perfluorocarbon gas or similar gases which have low solubility in blood and low diffusivity, providing extended echo-contrast enhancement.

MEDICAL APPLICATIONS OF ULTRASOUND CONTRAST AGENTS

This section provides a brief overview of how contrast agents are currently being used. It is meant to provide an understanding of the utility of the agents and indicate that, since there are many circumstances for their use now, it can be expected that additional applications may be found in obstetrics and gynecology which are not specifically identified here.

The use of ultrasound contrast agents began initially in echocardiography and provided increased echogenicity in the right chambers of the heart (i.e. not transpulmonary). As the agents have become more stable, their applica-tion has extended from the cardiac chambers to the myocardium, and include distal tissues such as the kidney, liver and brain (see review by Balens and co-workers[10]). In the heart, contrast agents have been used to assess shunts between heart chambers, dysfunctional valves and various congenital heart defects. Agents are now being visualized in the myocardium after intravenous injection, but the shorter boluses from intra-arterial injections of contrast agents have been used to assess myocardial perfusion, in which the intensity of the scattered sound is measured as a function of time as the agent passes through the tissue. Some contrast agents are now sufficiently stable to aid in evaluation of renal artery stenosis and renal blood flow assessment. Peripheral vascular detection of agents is now possible and tumor vascular studies are being performed on the basis of differences found in the neovasculature of malignant lesions. Blood pooling in the tumor provides for a prolonged enhancement by the contrast agent in tumor tissue.

Enhancement of Doppler signals may also provide a more accurate assessment of other flow characteristics said to be unique to cancer. Such studies have included the detection of hepatic lesions by Maresca and associates[25]. There have also been indications that thrombus may be better delineated by contrast agents due to an apparent affinity of the agent for the thrombus surface[26]. The signal enhancement from contrast agents can also help compensate for overlying attenuation in some Doppler examinations. A prime example is the use of contrast agents in cranial scanning. Effects of attenuation and aberration of the ultrasound field passing through the skull can be reduced substantially by the signal increase, which can be as much as 17 dB[27].

Non-vascular application

There are a number of non-vascular applications which are being developed for ultrasound contrast agents. These include some that are specifically related to obstetric and gynecological practice. The following is a brief description of some of these.

Hysterosalpingography has traditionally been performed using X-ray contrast to visualize uterine and pelvic pathology. Recently, however, ultrasound contrast examinations have compared favorably in many studies[28–30]. Ultrasound evaluations are made to detect uterine wall abnormalities such as endometrial polyps and submucosal fibroids. Fluid flow might also be used to determine Fallopian tube patency by monitoring flow into the pelvic cavity or using Doppler to detect the flow in the tube itself[29,31].

Urinary reflux has also been traditionally assessed using techniques which involve ionizing radiation. Experimental efforts with ultrasound contrast agents have indicated the potential to use an ultrasound contrast agent in such procedures. Specifically, two different agents have been examined for this purpose, Echovist and Albunex. In each case, the contrast agent has appeared in the kidney under known refluxing conditions. In addition, color Doppler has detected the movement of contrast in the ureters in canine experiments[32].

BUBBLE RESPONSE TO ULTRASOUND

Since most of the ultrasound contrast agents are based on gas bubbles, an understanding of the nature of the interaction of these bubbles with acoustic fields provides an understanding of how they work and their safety considerations. A gas bubble in a liquid such as water is a highly non-linear system, generating additional acoustic emissions owing to the large differences in density, sound speed and compressibility between the liquid and the gas. Non-linear bubble dynamics has been studied for many years and the subject has developed from research on the production of gas bubbles and their response to various stresses. The classic theoretical treatment of cavitation was the work of Lord Rayleigh[33], and was prompted by his desire to explain the sound made by boiling water and the cavitation produced by screw-propellers on ships. Since that time, a number of theoretical treatments of bubble interactions with sound have been derived and considerable effort has been made to understand the physical

consequences of cavitation[34]. Figure 1 shows theoretically how a free bubble and shelled bubble change their radii in response to the same acoustic field. The response of the shelled bubble is much less than that of the free bubble and therefore this might be less likely to produce a bioeffect. However, the apparent absence of free bubbles *in vivo* and the ability to introduce contrast agents may be more important in terms of the relative numbers of bubbles available to respond to the acoustic field and their potential as cavitation nuclei or 'seeds' for cavitation activity.

It is the response of the contrast agent to the acoustic field that provides the contrast enhancement seen in ultrasound images, and the non-linear nature of the response may be one of the reasons why contrast agents will be used even more in the future. When an acoustic field of a given frequency interacts with a contrast agent, the contrast agent responds by emitting not only the same frequency as the original acoustic field but also other frequencies (harmonics and subharmonics). For example, the bubble may produce an acoustic frequency twice that of the driver (termed a second harmonic). Some of these properties of contrast agents are being studied (harmonic imaging) and may further increase the utility of contrast agents. This is an area where safety of agents will need to be investigated, i.e. are agents driven to produce more harmonics more likely to produce bioeffects? The answers to many of these questions are, as yet, unknown.

Attenuation of the ultrasound due to the presence of bubbles can significantly reduce penetration and result in shadowing of underlying structures. A further consequence would be the local deposition of the acoustic energy into a reduced tissue volume. The non-linear conversion of acoustic energy to a higher frequency may be an area of future investigation.

SAFETY OF ULTRASOUND CONTRAST AGENTS

Bioeffect studies

For many years researchers interested in the effects of acoustic cavitation on biological

(a)

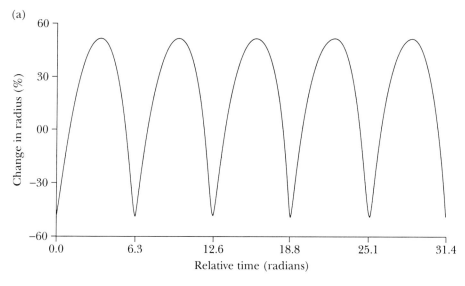

(b)

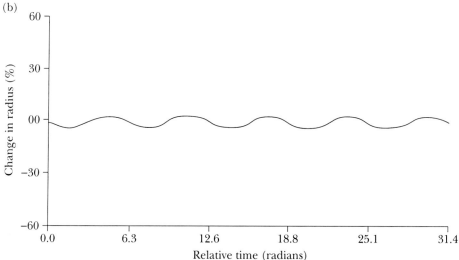

Figure 1 Radius–time curves for bubbles driven at 0.5 bars and 2 MHz, as modelled by the Keller-Herring equation for (a) a 1.7 μm radius resonant ideal gas bubble, and (b) a 4.8 μm radius resonant Albunex® microbubble including shell effects

systems have studied cavitation *in vivo*. Indications of damage have typically been at acoustic amplitudes which are high compared to the outputs from commercial diagnostic ultrasound systems except where gas pockets exist in tissue. Chapter 7 discusses the relevant issues associated with the likelihood of a cavitation event occurring particularly in the presence of free gas bubbles. One of the reasons why damage in *in vivo* systems has not been confirmed may be the absence of gas bubbles or cavitation nuclei needed as initiation points for acoustic cavitation. The introduction of a bubble-based contrast agent might change these conditions. As previously discussed, the shell that stabilizes the gas bubble against diffusion may also reduce the pulsation of the bubble and therefore lessen the effect of the bubble on the surrounding tissue. However, the added presence of gas bubbles in an otherwise bubble-free medium may be more important in determining the acoustic amplitude at which cavitation occurs, termed the cavitation threshold. Several *in vitro* and *in vivo* studies have been performed which examine the potential impact of contrast agents on the cavitation threshold, particularly in blood.

It has been known for some time that the presence of nuclei (stabilized pockets of gas) can greatly reduce the threshold for acoustic cavitation. Could the bubbles of some contrast agents do the same? The conclusions of experimental evidence varies as do the conditions under which the experiments were conducted. The following is a synopsis of a number of experiments in which contrast agents have been used as cavitation nuclei. First, the results in water are presented. These experiments provide the most direct indication of the sound–bubble interaction. However, these experiments lack some of the biological relevance of the results from *in vitro* and *in vivo* experiments. The *in vitro* results have concentrated around experiments in blood since the most common application for agents has been in vascular studies. Therefore, concern over the present use of ultrasound contrast agents in obstetric and gynecological applications is best discussed using results from both of these experimental situations.

Experimentation in cell-free media

Bioeffect studies of contrast agents have evolved to a great extent out of work that was already being conducted on the safety of diagnostic ultrasound. Several research groups around the world have been studying the potential effects of ultrasound interactions with biological systems and specifically the ability of ultrasound to produce cavitation. These experiments include work using various cavitation detection systems designed to monitor cavitation activity in aqueous media. Roy and colleagues[35] reported that the addition of Albunex reduced the cavitation threshold for filtered, degassed (~80% of saturation) water. In these experiments, the contrast agent was introduced into a tank of filtered, deionized, degassed water. The agent then passed through the beam of a 1.0- or 2.25-MHz transducer producing 10 μs tone

bursts at 1 kHz pulse repetition frequency. The rapid expansion of a cavitation event at the focus scatters the transmitted field which is detected by a second transducer (termed passive detection). When the 1-MHz field was used, little or no cavitation was reported at acoustic pressure amplitudes below 0.25–0.30 MPa. The rate of cavitation increased steadily up to 0.5–0.6 MPa, at which point a cavitation event occurred every time a contrast agent bubble entered the focus of the field. At 2.25 MHz, cavitation activity was detected at amplitudes above 0.3–0.35 MPa. However, even at 1.0 MPa, 30–50% of the bubbles passed through the focus without initiating a cavitation event.

Holland and Apfel[36] presented results of experiments using a similar passive detection system in which frequencies of 0.757, 0.989 and 2.300 MHz were tested. Experiments used different materials as cavitation nuclei including 1 μm diameter polystyrene spheres, approximately 4 μm Albunex and red blood cells. The host medium was water, 80% ethylene glycol in water, or isotonic saline, all of which were filtered (0.25 μm) and degassed (approximately 50% of saturation). The cavitation threshold for pure water ranged from 2.0 to 4.0 MPa. A jet of fluid was used to convect the nuclei through the focus of the ultrasonic beam. The threshold was 1.94–2.43 MPa with a jet of filtered, degassed water, and this value increased slightly with increasing acoustic frequency. In experiments with a dilute solution of Albunex in the jet only one frequency, 0.757 MHz, was used. The threshold was reduced from 1.59 MPa when the jet contained only 5% albumin solution to 0.52–0.64 MPa when the contrast agent was included. This is a substantial reduction in threshold, greater than that seen with the polystyrene spheres. The threshold for filtered, degassed saline ranged from 1.39 to 1.85 MPa and the authors noted that this range might be due to differences in fluid handling. The addition of dilute solutions of red blood cells did not change the threshold found in saline. Holland and associates[37] also performed experiments using a 30-MHz pulse-echo system (active cavitation detector)[38] to detect cavitation. A Hewlett-Packard 77020A diagnostic ultrasound system was used to produce cavitation and Albunex provided the cavitation nuclei when introduced into filtered (0.2 mm), degassed (50–60% of saturation) water. Operating in both the M-mode (single cycle) and pulsed Doppler (four cycles), no cavitation activity was detected when the contrast agent was injected into the focus at pressure amplitudes up to 1.3 and 1.2 MPa for frequencies of 2.5 and 5.0 MHz, respectively. However, the author expressed reservations concerning the sensitivity of the detector to cavitation events due to the large scattering measured at 30 MHz from the contrast agent itself.

Other studies have used the production of hydrogen peroxide (H_2O_2) as an indicator of inertial cavitation[39]. During inertial cavitation, bubble collapse is driven by the inertia of the liquid and results in elevated temperatures and pressures within the bubble. Such collapse conditions have been shown to produce free radical chemistry and the end result is the production of H_2O_2. In these experiments filtered phosphate-buffered saline was introduced into a culture tube which could be rotated at a fixed rate. The tube was then exposed to ultrasound at frequencies of 2.17, 2.95, or 3.8 MHz. When dilute solutions of either Albunex or Levovist were included in the saline, significant H_2O_2 production was measured at acoustic amplitudes of 0.41 MPa or higher at 2.17 MHz frequency. The exposures were 5 min in duration with 0.25-s burst lengths and a 1 : 2 duty cycle which is not generally representative of diagnostic exposures. The tube rotated at 60 rpm; if the tube was stationary, the H_2O_2 production was virtually eliminated. For 2.5-min continuous exposures, both agents produced significant H_2O_2 at an acoustic pressure threshold amplitude of 0.58 MPa for 2.95-MHz fields, but not at amplitudes up to 1.16 MPa for 3.8-MHz fields.

In summary, contrast agents do appear to act as cavitation nuclei in cell-free aqueous media under certain circumstances. One item of note is the repeated use of degassed solutions. The reduced gas content in the host medium may adversely affect some contrast agents (Harold Levene, personal communication,

and our laboratory experiences with Albunex). Although some bubbles may persist in the liquid as evidenced by an increased scattering of the acoustic field after injection, the bubbles may be altered and may not respond as they would without the effects of the reduced gas content in the liquid. There is some tendency, at least among the studies described above, for the contrast agents to be less efficient as cavitation nuclei at higher frequencies and perhaps shorter burst lengths. Therefore, one might anticipate a greater potential for cavitation using Doppler pulses and a reduced risk at the higher frequencies commonly used in diagnostic imaging. However, the peak negative pressure produced by diagnostic ultrasound imaging systems is typically higher in non-Doppler modes. Results from Holland and Apfel[36] indicated that the cavitation threshold remains high in saline even with the addition of cells at low concentrations. Increasing the viscosity of the medium theoretically increases the cavitation threshold[40], but this was not supported by the experiments described.

Experimentation in biological media

Several *in vitro* studies indicate that cavitation thresholds decrease with the introduction of microbubbles within sample fluids that have a low particle or cell count; these test fluids effectively have viscosities of the same order as water. Using the HL-60 human promyelocytic leukemia cell line at a concentration of 8×10^5 cells/ml, Jeffers and associates[41] added an aliquot of 5% bovine albumin solution and showed no cell lysis at intensities of 2.5 W/cm^2 with 1 MHz continuous wave ultrasound. However, when the same amount of sonicated albumin microbubbles was introduced to the sample fluid, cells began to lyse at 1 W/cm^2 and lysis increased with increasing intensity, to a level of about 35% at 2.5 W/cm^2.

Brayman and co-workers[42] and Miller and associates[43] studied cavitation in blood at varying hematocrits. Brayman and colleagues used 1.1 MHz high-intensity pulsed ultrasound (8.5 W/cm^2 I_{SPTA}) to show, in the absence of Albunex, that there was no red blood cell lysis, except at 1% hematocrit, whereas when Albunex was added to the sample blood, cell lysis occurred at all hematocrits tested. Miller and colleagues[43] performed several combinations of experiments to show that with 1 MHz continuous wave ultrasound from 0 to 5 W/cm^2, low hematocrit samples, at < 20%, were significantly affected by the addition of Albunex, resulting in more hemolysis in general with increasing intensity. Similarly, Williams and co-workers[44] found that hemolysis decreased with increasing hematocrit with Echovist present, and that no hemolysis was detected at hematocrits of 5.5% and greater, with 0.75 MHz continuous wave ultrasound at intensities as high as 3 W/cm^2.

More clinically and physiologically relevant results in vascular applications are those studies done with whole blood (about 40% hematocrit in humans). Continuous wave ultrasound at 1 MHz was not shown to lyse red blood cells in whole blood with Albunex at intensities up to 5 W/cm^2 [43]. In contrast, Brayman and co-workers[42] found significant hemolysis in whole blood containing Albunex using high-intensity pulses (8.5 W/cm^2 I_{SPTA}). However, these studies used continuous wave ultrasound or conditions that produced average intensities nearer to therapeutic than diagnostic applications.

To support the safety results of using higher doses of Albunex, Miller and associates[43] showed in an in vitro experiment that for all concentrations between 1.3 μl/ml and 40 μl/ml, the same amount of hemolysis was seen in blood samples at 1% hematocrit, when exposed to 1 MHz continuous wave ultrasound at 5 W/cm^2. The finding that hemolysis was independent of Albunex® concentration suggests that cell lysis saturation occurs at very low concentrations.

The mechanical index (MI), formulated by the AIUM/NEMA[45] as a predictor of non-thermal mechanical effects of ultrasound, is intended to determine the likelihood of substantial inertial cavitation in the presence of diagnostic ultrasound[46]. The MI weights the peak pressure expected with the frequency of operation to the properties of the host fluid and a value less than 0.5 indicates small likelihood that cavitation will occur, however, values above

0.5 indicate that larger amounts of bubble activity can be expected. In the theoretical development of this index, analytic and numeric studies showed the influence of fluid inertia, viscosity and surface tension on the damping of growth of a bubble and subsequent pulsation, thereby decreasing the potential for cavitation. With whole blood having a viscosity five times that of water ($\mu_{water} = 1 \times 10^{-3}$ N/m and $\mu_{blood} = 5 \times 10^{-3}$ N/m), the calculated mechanical index for identical exposure conditions is expected to be lower for blood than for water.

It should be understood that these in vitro results have relevance to the in vivo case only when the mechanism for bioeffects can be reasonably expected and that the final test will be the determination that such effects are demonstrated in vivo. There is some evidence that the threshold for cavitation bioeffects is reduced in the presence of Albunex[47]. Hemolysis was observed in various tissue types exposed to ultrasound, only after injection of the contrast agent. The authors believed that the agent was acting as cavitation nuclei. In addition, the disappearance of contrast agent in the presence of diagnostic levels of ultrasound has not only been reported in vivo, but has actually developed into a research area termed transient response imaging in which the frame rate of the ultrasound imaging system is purposefully kept low to reduce the disappearance of contrast enhancement[48,49]. One agent, Cavisomes® (Schering AG) is designed to be taken up into the reticuloendothelial system and collapse in the presence of diagnostic ultrasound to produce transient Doppler shifts due to induced acoustic emissions. It is uncertain whether these contrast agents can be disrupted without biological consequence.

The mechanical index makes a distinction between situations with and without the known presence of gas bodies thought to enhance the probability for mechanical effects. Further research is needed to determine whether contrast agents will affect the selection of MI limits.

The World Federation for Ultrasound in Medicine and Biology (WFUMB) recently held an international symposium on safety of ultrasound in medicine[50]. WFUMB has issued a recommendation on the use of echo-contrast agents which states:

> Gas bodies introduced by a contrast agent increase the probability of cavitation. A physician should take this into account when considering the benefit/risk ratio of an examination.

Clinical studies

The two agents that have been used extensively in clinical trials are Albunex and Levovist, because of their stability and ability to traverse the pulmonary vasculature. Initial concerns about the use of gas-filled stabilized microbubbles involved the possibility that they could obstruct the capillaries of organs, including the brain. However, several reports have concluded that gas microbubbles are relatively safe in this respect[51,52]. Also, since the mean bubble sizes of Albunex and Levovist and newer bubble contrast agents are approximately 3 μm in diameter, these agents will either pass through these capillary beds, or quickly dissolve.

In the case of Echovist and Levovist (SH U 454 and 508 A, respectively), the suspended galactose microparticles will gradually dissolve after injection into the blood. Levovist differs from Echovist in that it also contains a fatty acid that stabilizes the microparticle for longer contrast enhancement. Extensive clinical experience with Echovist (> 1850 patients for echocardiography, > 200 for venous vessels and > 500 for hysterosalpingocontrast sonography) and Levovist (> 200 for echocardiography) has not shown significant adverse clinical effects[25,53].

To eliminate the use of ionizing or iodinated contrast agents for gynecological examinations, several investigators have used saline as a negative contrast medium to aid in ultrasound imaging of uterine and extrauterine structures[28,30,31]. This imaging method, dubbed sonosalpingography by one investigator, has been shown to be sensitive for diagnosing uterine pathology[30] and effective in indirectly diagnosing unilateral Fallopian tube patency[28,31,54]. With the indications of the mechanical index and results from the *in vitro* blood studies, it would seem efficacious from a bioeffects standpoint perhaps to use a more viscous fluid than saline, whose viscosity is similar to that of water, for these examinations, if microbubbles are to be introduced and exposed to ultrasound. However, from the clinical study by Richman and colleagues[28], the use of Hyskon, a highly viscous fluid, caused more discomfort to the patient and did not flow as easily as saline.

Human albumin solutions are widely used for plasma expansion and other blood applications. Decades of clinical use in these areas have shown a low occurrence of adverse effects. Because Albunex is generated from sonicated human albumin and is also suspended in a 5% (w/v) albumin solution, concern had arisen over possible adverse immunogenic reactions. Also, Ostensen and co-workers[55] observed that injection of Albunex caused pulmonary hypertension in pigs, but not in monkeys or rabbits. It is believed that this reaction is due to species-related pulmonary morphology[56]. However, in two experiments in which Albunex was injected into healthy subjects, no evidence was found that this microbubble would invoke an adverse immunological response even after repeated exposure to Albunex[57,58]. In an investigation of the washout of Albunex after injection, it was found that after 3 min 80% of the injected agent was retained in the liver. The microspheres are then phagocytized by the reticuloendothelial system, and the waste by-products are flushed from the body through the urine[59].

To answer the question of safety and efficacy of use of ultrasound contrast agents, Geny and colleagues[60] studied the effect of Albunex injections on systemic and pulmonary hemodynamics of patients with ischemic heart disease. Two injection doses were administered to determine whether opacification of the left ventricle increased enough to justify giving the higher dosage of contrast agent. Results showed that, in all patients, no immediate or delayed adverse hemodynamic or respiratory changes were recorded, and the higher dosage of Albunex gave a 20% increase in observed opacification. Similarly, ten Cate and co-workers[61] measured no changes in left ventricular hemodynamics when Albunex was administered intracoronarily to patients with stable coronary artery disease.

Table 1 Selected observations concerning the use and bioeffects of Albunex® and Echovist®/Levovist®

Agent	Type/constitution	In vitro experiments	In vivo clinical results
Albunex	microbubble with albumin shell	Brayman et al. (1995)[42] RBC lysis in whole blood using high-intensity pulsed ultrasound (8.5 W/cm² SPTA)	Christiansen et al. (1994)[57] no evidence of adverse immunological reaction with intravenous administration
		Miller et al. (1995)[43] no RBC lysis in whole blood using continuous wave ultrasound 0–5 W/cm²	Wible et al. (1994)[12] study under way for use in FTP tests
		Holland et al. (1992)[37] no cavitation observed in water using diagnostic frequencies and intensities (M-mode and Doppler mode)	Geny et al. (1993)[60] no clinical, hemodynamic or respiratory adverse reactions in patients with ischemic heart disease
		Holland and Apfel (1990)[36] lowered cavitation threshold in water from 16 to 6 atm at 0.757 MHz	ten Cate et al. (1993)[61] no change in measured left-heart hemodynamics in patients with stable coronary artery disease, with intra-coronary injection
			Feinstein et al. (1990)[62] multicenter study – no serious side-effects of intravenous administration; minor adverse effects noted, but brief and quickly and naturally resolved
Saline	(negative contrast)	Holland and Apfel (1990)[36] cavitation threshold for saline similar to threshold for water (~16 atm)	Balen et al. (1993)[31] effective indirect method over ultrasound alone or Echovist in FTP testing
			Bonilla-Musoles et al. (1992)[30] saline ultrasound contrast HSG more sensitive over hysteroscopy for diagnosis of uterine pathologies
			Richman et al. (1984)[28] more effective than conventional FTP testing
Echovist/ Levovist	galactose microparticle/ with added fatty acid	Williams et al. (1991)[44] no RBC lysis in whole blood with continuous wave ultrasound at intensities as high as 3 W/cm²	Maresca et al. (1994)[25] Levovist effective in delineating focal hepatic lesions
			Balen et al. (1993)[31] not reliable in diagnosis of tubal patency; 20% of patients complained of mild discomfort
			Schlief et al. (1993)[53] review of clinical use shows no relevant changes in cardiovascular function, no substance-induced severe adverse effects
			Schlief and Deichert (1991)[29] improved diagnostic accuracy in tubal patency tests using B- and Doppler modes; agent well tolerated by patients

RBC, red blood cells; FTP, Fallopian tube patency test; HSG, hysterosalpingography

In a multicenter study of healthy patients, with some having only mild hypertension, Feinstein and colleagues[62] injected Albunex intravenously to determine the safety of its use and to evaluate its ability to opacify the left chambers of the heart. All 71 patients, some of whom had multiple injections, had good tolerance to the agent and showed no significant changes in clinical variables, such as electrocardiogram, physical or neurological abnormalities. A few patients were noted to have experienced mild, temporary adverse reactions ranging from lightheadedness to erythema near the injection site.

Additional clinical experiences with both Albunex and Levovist indicate that other minor reactions to intravenous injections include a mild feeling of generalized warmth or coolness in the injected arm (Jonathan Rubin, personal communication).

General results have been that no significant/functional adverse physiological reactions have occurred in these human studies and that the agents were well tolerated by the subjects. Table 1 summaries the *in vitro* and *in vivo* work for the more commonly used contrast agents in clinical settings.

References

1. Gramiak, R., Shah, P. M. and Kramer, D.H. (1969). Ultrasound cardiography: contrast studies in anatomy and function. *Radiology*, **92**, 939–48
2. Ziskin, M. C., Bonakdapour, A., Wienstein, D. P. and Lynch, P. R. (1972). Contrast agents for diagnostic ultrasound. *Invest. Radiol.*, **6**, 500–5
3. Meltzer, R. S., Tickner, E., Sahines, T. and Popp, R. L. (1980). The source of ultrasound contrast effect. *J. Clin. Ultrasound*, **8**, 121–7
4. Ophir, J. and Parker, K. J. (1989). Contrast agents in diagnostic ultrasound. *Ultrasound Med. Biol.*, **15**, 319–33
5. Meerbaum, S. and Meltzer, R. S. (1989). *Myocardial Contrast Two-Dimensional Echocardiography*. (The Netherlands: Kluwer Academic Press)
6. de Jong, N. (1991). Principles and recent developments in ultrasound contrast agents. [Review]. *Ultrasonics*, **29**, 324–30
7. Mattrey, R. and Steinbach, G. (1991). Ultrasound contrast agents. State of the art. [Review]. *Invest. Radiol.*, **26** (Suppl. 1), S5–S11
8. Goldberg, B. B., Liu, J. B. and Forsberg, F. (1994). Ultrasound contrast agents: a review. *Ultrasound Med. Biol.*, **20**, 319–33
9. Winkelmann, J. W., Kenner, M. D., Dave, R., Chandwaney, R. H. and Feinstein, S. B. (1994). Contrast echocardiography. *Ultrasound Med. Biol.*, **20**, 507–15
10. Balen, F. G., Allen, C. M. and Lees, W. R. (1994). Ultrasound contrast agents. *Clin. Radiol.*, **49**, 77–82
11. Burns, P. (1994). Ultrasound contrast agents in radiological diagnosis. [Review]. *Radiol. Med.*, **87** (5 Suppl. 1), 71–82
12. Wible, J. H., Adams, M. D., Sherwin, P. F., Wojdyla, J. K., Parsons, A. K., Atala, A., Fowlkes, J. B. and Needleman, L. (1994). Noncardiac applications of Albunex®. *Invest. Radiol.*, **29** (Suppl. 2), S145–8
13. Harvey, E. N., Barnes, K. K., McElroy, W. D., Whitely, A. H., Pease, D. C. and Cooper, K. W. J. (1944). Bubble formation in animals, I. Physical factors. *J. Cell Comp. Physiol.*, **21**, 1–22
14. Crum, L. (1979). Tensile strength in water. *Nature (London)*, **278**, 148–9
15. Yount, D. E. (1979). Skins of varying permeability: a stabilization mechanism for gas cavitation nuclei. *J. Acoust. Soc. Am.*, **65**, 1429–39
16. Carroll, B., Turner, R., Tichner, E. and SW, Y. (1980). Microbubbles as ultrasonic contrast agents. *Invest. Radiol.*, **15**, 260–6
17. Feinstein, S. B., Keller, M. W. and Kerber, R. E. (1989). Sonicated echocardiographic contrast agents: reproducibility studies. *J. Am. Coll. Cardiol.*, **2**, 125–31
18. Smith, M. D., Kwan, O. L., Reisner, H. J. and DeMaria, A. N. (1984). Superior intensity and reproducibility of ShU-454, a new right heart contrast agent. *J. Am. Coll. Cardiol.*, **3**, 992–8
19. Simon, R. H., Ho, S. Y., D'Arrigo, J. S., Wakefield, A. E. and Hamilton, S. (1990). Lipid-coated microbubbles as a contrast agent in neurosonography. *Invest. Radiol.*, **25**, 1300–4
20. Unger, E. C., Lund, P. J., Fritz, T. A., Fuller, E. and Tilcock, C. (1990). Aerosomes liposome as ultrasound contrast agent. *Radiology*, **181(P)**, 225 (abstr.)
21. Unger, E. C., Lund, P. J., Shen, D.-K. and Fritz, T. A. (1992). Nitrogen-filled liposomes as a

vascular ultrasound contrast agent: preliminary evaluation. *Radiology*, **185**, 453–6

22. de Jong, N., ten Cate, F. J., Vletter, W. B. and Roelancts, J. (1993). Quantification of transpulmonary echo-contrast effects. *Ultrasound Med. Biol.*, **19**, 279–88

23. Parker, K., Tuthill, T., Lerner, R. and Violante, M. (1987). A particulate contrast agent with potential for ultrasound imaging of liver. *Ultrasound Med. Biol.*, **13**, 555–66

24. Needleman, L., Merton, D. A., Liu, J. B. and Goldberg, B. B. (1995). Evaluation of the safety and contrast enhancement of intravenous Echo-Gen® in normal adult males. *J. Ultrasound Med.*, **14**, S55 (abstr.)

25. Maresca, G., Barbaro, B., Summaria, V., De-Gaetano, A. M., Salcuni, M., Mirk, P. and Marano, P. (1994). Color Doppler ultrasonography in the differential diagnosis of focal hepatic lesions. The SH U 508 A (Levovist) experience. *Radiol. Med.*, **87**(Suppl. 1), 41–9

26. Needleman, L., Nack, T. L., Feld, R. I. and Goldberg, B. B. (1992). Initial experience with an ultrasound contrast agent in upper-extremity venous thrombosis. *Radiology*, **185(P)**, 143 (abstr.)

27. Rosenkranz, K., Zendel, W., Langer, R., Heim, T., Schubeus, P., Scholz, A., Schlief, R., Schurmann, R. and Felix, R. (1993). Contrast-enhanced transcranial Doppler US with a new transpulmonary echo contrast agent based on saccharide microparticles. *Radiology*, **187**, 439–43

28. Richman, T. S., Viscomi, G. N., de Cherney, A., Polan, M. and Alcébo, L. O. (1984). Fallopian tubal patency assessed by ultrasound following fluid injections. *Radiology*, **152**, 507–10

29. Schief, R. and Deichert, U. (1991). Hysterosalpingo-contrast sonography of the uterus and fallopian tubes: results of a clinical trial with a new ultrasound contrast medium in 120 patients. *Radiology*, **178**, 213–15

30. Bonilla-Musoles, F., Simon, C., Serra, V., Sampaio, M. and Pellicer, A. (1992). An assessment of hysterosalpingosonography (HSSG) as a diagnostic tool for uterine cavity defects and tubal patency. *J. Clin. Ultrasound*, **20**, 175–81

31. Balen, F. G., Allen, C. M., Siddle, N. C. and Lees, W. R. (1993). Ultrasound contrast hysterosalpingography evaluation as an outpatient procedure. *Br. J. Radiol.*, **66**, 592–9

32. Ivey, J. A., Fowlkes, J. B., Gardner, E. A., Feitz, W. F. J., Bloom, D. A., Carson, P. L. and Rubin, J. M. (1993). *In vivo* observation of urinary reflux using ultrasound contrast agents. In *1993 Annual Meeting, Association of University Radiologists*, Cincinnati, OH, May 19–23 (abstr.)

33. Rayleigh, L. (1917). On the pressure developed in a liquid during the collapse of a spherical cavity. *Phil. Mag.*, **34**, 94

34. Leighton, T. G. (1994). Effects and mechanism. In *The Acoustic Bubble*, pp.539–90 (London: Academic Press)

35. Roy, R. A., Church, C. C. and Calabrese, A. (1990). Cavitation produced by short pulses of ultrasound. In *Frontiers in Nonlinear Acoustics: Proceedings of 12th ISNA*, Austin, TX, pp. 476–81. (London: Elsevier Science Publishers)

36. Holland, C. K. and Apfel, R. E. (1990). Thresholds for transient cavitation produced by pulsed ultrasound in a controlled nuclei environment. *J. Acoust. Soc. Am.*, **88**, 2059–69

37. Holland, C. K., Roy, R. A., Apfel, R. E. and Crum, L. A. (1992). *In vitro* detection of cavitation induced by a diagnostic ultrasound system. *IEEE Trans. UFFC*, **39**, 95–101

38. Roy, R. A., Madanshetty, S. and Apfel, R. E. (1990). An acoustic backscattering technique for the detection of transient cavitation produced by microsecond pulses of ultrasound. *J. Acoust. Soc. Am.*, **87**, 2451–5

39. Miller, D. L. and Thomas, R. M. (1996). Role of cavitation in the induction of cellular DNA damage by ultrasound and lithotripter shock waves *in vitro*. *Ultrasound Med. Biol.*, **22**, 681–7

40. Holland, C. K. and Apfel, R. E. (1989). An improved theory for the prediction of microcavitation due to pulsed ultrasound. *IEEE Trans. UFFC*, **36**, 204–8

41. Jeffers, R. J., Feng, R. Q., Fowlkes, J. B., Hunt, J. W., Kessel, D. and Cain, C. A. (1995). Dimethylformamide as an enhancer of cavitation-induced cell lysis *in vitro*. *J. Acoust. Soc. Am.*, **97**, 669–76

42. Brayman, A. A., Azadniv, M., Makin, I. R. S., Miller, M. W., Carstensen, E. L., Child, S. Z., Raeman, C. H., Meltzer, R. S. and Everbach, E. C. (1995). Effect of a stabilized microbubble echo contrast agent on hemolysis of human erythrocytes exposed to high intensity pulsed ultrasound. *Echocardiography*, **12**, 13–21

43. Miller, M. W., Azadniv, M. and Doida, Y. (1995). Effect of a stabilized microbubble contrast agent on CW ultrasound induced red blood cell lysis *in vitro*. *Echocardiography*, **12**, 1–11

44. Williams, A., Kubowicz, G., Cramer, E. and Schlief, R. (1991). The effects of the microbubble suspension SH U 454 (Echovist®) on ultrasound-induced cell lysis in a rotating tube exposure system. *Echocardiography*, **8**, 423–33

45. American Institute of Ultrasound in Medicine (1992). *Standard for Real-time Display of Thermal and Mechanical Acoustic Indices on Diagnostic Ultrasound Equipment.* (Laurel, MD: AIUM)

46. Apfel, R. E. and Holland, C. K. (1991). Guaging the likelihood of cavitation from short-pulse, low-duty cycle diagnostic ultrasound. *Ultrasound Med. Biol.*, **17**, 179–85

47. Carstensen, E. L. (1996). Biological effects on tissues containing stabilized bubbles. *J. Ultrasound Med.*, **15** (Suppl.), S24

48. Sirlin, Girard, M. S., Baker, K., Hall, L. A., Steinbach, R. F. and Mattrey, R. F. (1996). Effect of gated US acquisition on liver and portal vein contrast enhancement. *Radiology*, **201P**, 195

49. Moriyasu, F., Kono, Y., Nada, T., Matsumura, T., Suginoshita, Y. and Kobayashi, K. (1996). Flash echo (passive cavitation) imaging of the liver by using US contrast agents and intermittent scanning sequence. *Radiology*, **201P**, 196

50. Barnett, S. B. (ed.) (1997). Conclusions and recommendations on thermal and non-thermal mechanisms for biological effects of ultrasound. In *World Federation for Ultrasound in Medicine and Biology Symposium on Safety of Ultrasound In Medicine. Ultrasound Med. Biol.*, in press

51. Bommer, W., Shah, P., Allen, H., Meltzer, R. and Kisslo, J. (1984). *Contrast Echocardiography.* Report for the American Society of Echocardiography, pp. 1–10

52. Gillam, L., Kaul, S., Fallon, J. T., Levine, R. A., Hedley-Whyte, E. T., Guerrero, J. L. and Weyman, A. E. (1984). Functional and pathologic effects of multiple echocardio-graphic contrast injections on the myocardium, brain and kidney. *J. Am. Coll. Cardiol.*, **6**, 687–94

53. Schlief, R., Schurman, R. and Niendorf, H.P. (1993). Basic properties and results of clinical trials of ultrasound contrast agents based on galactose. *Ann. Acad. Med.*, **22**, 762–7

54. Randolph, J. R., Ying, Y. K., Maier, D. B., Schmidt, C. L. and Riddick, D. H. (1986). Comparison of real-time ultrasonography hysterosalpingography, and laparoscopy/hysteroscopy in the evaluation of uterine abnormalities and tubal patency. *Fertil. Steril.*, **46**, 828–32

55. Ostensen, J., Hede, R., Myreng, Y., Ege, T. and Holtz, E. (1992). Intravenous injection of Albunex® microspheres causes thromboxane mediated pulmonary hypertension in pigs, but not in monkeys or rabbits. *ACC Acta Physiol. Scand.*, **144**, 307–15

56. DeCamp, M. M., Warner, A. E., Molina, R. M. and Brain, J. D. (1992). Hepatic versus pulmonary uptake of particles injected into the portal circulation in sheep. Endotoxin escapes hepatic clearance causing pulmonary inflammation. *Am. Rev. Respir. Dis.*, **146**, 224–31

57. Christiansen, C., Vebner, A. J., Muan, B., Vik, H., Haider, T., Nicolaysen, H. and Skotland, T. (1994). Lack of an immune response to Albunex®, a new ultrasound contrast agent based on air-filled albumin microspheres. *Int. Arch. Allergy Immunol.*, **104**, 372–8

58. Barnhart, J. L., Harada, M., Lyle, L. R. and Saravis, C. A. (1991). Immunologic reactions of human recipients to repeated exposures to Albunex® microspheres. *Invest. Radiol.*, **26**, S192–3

59. Keller, M., Glasheen, W. and Kaul, S. (1989). Albunex®: a safe and effective commercially produced agent for myocardial contrast echocardiography. *J. Am. Soc. Echocardiol.*, **2**, 48–52

60. Geny, B., Mettauer, B., Muan, B., Bischoff, P., Epailly, E., Piquard, F., Eisenmann, B. and Haberey, P. (1993). Safety and efficacy of a new transpulmonary echo-contrast agent in echocardiographic studies in patients. *Am. Coll. Cardiol.*, **22**, 1193–8

61. Ten-Cate, F. J., Widimsky, P., Cornel, J. H., Waldstein, D. J., Serruys, P. W. and Waaler, A. (1993). Intracoronary Albunex®: its effects on left ventricular hemodynamics, function, and coronary sinus flow in humans. *Circulation*, **88**, 2123–7

62. Feinstein, S. B., Cheirif, J., Ten Cate, F. J., Silverman, P. R., Heidenreich, P. A., Dick, C., Desir, R. M., Arstrong, W. F., Quinones, M. A. and Shah, P. M. (1990). Safety and efficacy of a new transpulmonary ultrasound contrast agent: initial multicenter clinical results. *J. Am. Coll. Cardiol.*, **16**, 316–24

Acoustic streaming and radiation pressure in diagnostic applications: what are the implications?

9

F. A. Duck

SUMMARY

Low-level radiation stresses (forces) are always exerted on the tissues of both mother and fetus by the pulses of ultrasound used in ultrasonic scanning. These forces are sufficient to cause fluid to flow away from the transducer along the path of the ultrasound beam, within volumes of at least 1 ml. There is no evidence of hazard associated with this streaming when generated within amniotic fluid or urine. Within soft tissues the radiation stress is probably insufficient to cause gross damage at diagnostic intensities, although the effect of stress enhancement near large acoustic boundaries requires further study. Radiation pressure from ultrasonic pulses of diagnostic amplitude, but longer duration, has been shown to cause compression ischemia, and can be sensed by the skin. Weakly tethered cell structures, and in particular embryonic tissue, could bear the risk of disturbance if the recovery from the application of a transient stress wave were incomplete. Any decision to use diagnostic ultrasound during the first trimester should acknowledge radiation stress as a potential bioeffects mechanism and, prudently, reduced exposure levels should be used.

INTRODUCTION

The mechanisms of tissue heating and acoustic cavitation have both been given considerable attention as ultrasound safety issues. The physical processes in each case have been subject to extensive theoretical analysis, and there is some experimental validation of theoretical predictions. There is also a reasonable understanding of the biological impact of heating and cavitation when they occur in living tissue. These issues are addressed elsewhere in this volume. This chapter describes another physical process that needs proper attention for appreciation of the possible biological consequences of the passage of ultrasound through tissue. A number of forces act directly on the tissue when ultrasound passes through. Whilst these forces are themselves generally small, there are some conditions in which their effects can be readily perceived. In particular, when ultrasound passes through a liquid, the liquid is pushed along by the beam, causing it to 'stream' in the direction along the path of the beam away from the transducer. Acoustic streaming has been known since the 19th century, having been observed by Faraday[1] in the air above vibrating plates in 1831. When liquids are exposed to diagnostic ultrasound beams under appropriate conditions, streaming can occur, and this has been observed both in laboratory experiments, and also *in vivo*. With this evidence to hand it is possible to speculate with greater understanding about the possible biological reaction to the acoustic radiation forces exerted within the body. The forces that cause streaming also act throughout all the tissues through which an ultrasound beam passes, and whilst it is true that generally no permanent deformation of soft tissue will occur, there are some circumstances when weakly bound tissue might be affected. Examples of such weak tissues are those within the embryo, the eye and the

---

brain. The present state of knowledge in this relatively unexplored area of ultrasound safety is the subject of the present chapter.

RADIATION STRESSES IN DIAGNOSTIC BEAMS

Radiation force

Before consideration of the general question of radiation forces exerted throughout a three-dimensional medium, a rather simpler example is discussed. A solid object placed in an ultrasound beam propagating in a liquid experiences a range of forces[2], of which the simplest example is that due to energy transfer from the wave. This force tends to push the object away from the transducer. The strength of the 'push' depends on relatively few factors: the size of the object in comparison with the beam, whether it reflects or absorbs ultrasound, the angle and shape of the front surface of the object and, finally, the intensity or power of the ultrasound beam.

When the object is larger than the ultrasound beam the total *radiation force* depends on the total acoustic power in the beam. Careful measurement of this force forms the basis of a standard method of measuring acoustic power[3]. For an object that completely absorbs the beam energy, the force in newtons (F) is given simply by the ratio of the power in watts (W) to the velocity of ultrasound in the liquid in meters per second (c):

$$F = W/c$$

This force is not very large. For a beam with a total acoustic power of 1 W (a little higher than the greatest power used for Doppler applications, see Chapter 3) the force is approximately equivalent to a weight of a 69-mg mass, if the liquid is water. If the surface of the object is a total reflector perpendicular to the beam, rather than a total absorber, the force is twice this amount. In both cases the total force results from a local stress acting perpendicularly to every point on the surface of the object which is in the ultrasound beam. This stress is called the *radiation pressure*. Note that the radiation pressure does not vary at the ultrasonic frequency,

and is distinct from the oscillating *acoustic pressure* of the ultrasonic wave.

Radiation pressure

The purpose of the present discussion is not simply to consider the macroscopic forces on large objects, but also to explore in more detail the way these forces, more strictly the radiation stresses, operate on the tissue being traversed by an ultrasonic pulse, and what the outcome might be on the structures subject to such stresses. To this end the complexity will be developed a step at a time. Next we shall consider the stress profile at the surface of a fully absorbing barrier across a typical ultrasonic diagnostic beam, with a beamwidth of a few millimeters. The radiation pressure varies with the ultrasonic beam intensity profile at the interface. The local radiation pressure (P) exerted on a totally absorbing surface is simply the ratio between the local time-averaged intensity (I) and acoustic velocity (c):

$$P = I/c$$

A radiation pressure profile can therefore be calculated from an independent measurement of the beam intensity profile; an example is shown in Figure 1, using a typical focal beam intensity profile of a pulsed Doppler beam. This illustrates the variation of the stress across the beam, being greatest on the beam axis and reducing towards its boundary. It may be compared with the effect of a blunt point on a

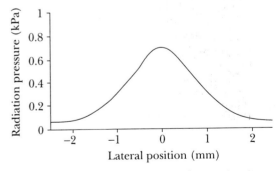

Figure 1 Radiation pressure profile at the focus during a diagnostic pulse, on an absorbing surface, $I_{SPPA} = 100$ W/cm^2

surface. Whilst the prediction of internal stresses resulting from this external pressure distribution is complex, one known outcome is the generation of shear forces within the solid. The degree of shear will depend on the material properties of the object and on the magnitude of the applied stress. It also depends on the gradient of radiation pressure across the beam. Thus a full judgement concerning the potential significance of these stresses must take account of not only the peak radiation pressure, calculated from the peak intensity, but also the beamwidth, and hence the radial rate of change of the forward stress across the beam.

Radiation pressure gradient

The next level of complexity is to consider what happens, not simply at an interface, but throughout the three-dimensional volume of insonated tissue. In general any attenuating substance experiences internal forces in the direction of ultrasound propagation as a result of energy lost from the beam to the medium. The term 'radiation pressure' is strictly defined only for an interface, and should therefore not be used to describe the local internal stress within a material, although the term has been so used from time to time. Strictly the term *radiation stress tensor* should be used[4]. Irrespective of the terminology, the important concept is that when an ultrasound beam travels through an absorbing material (such as soft tissue) it experiences an internal force throughout the material in the direction of the wave. The local strength can be calculated if the *in situ* intensity is known; in this case the *radiation stress gradient* along the wave (assuming it is a plane wave) is $2\alpha I/c$, where α is the attenuation coefficient, and c is the acoustic velocity. The unit of measurement is Pa/mm. (At times in the literature this is referred to as the *radiation pressure gradient*[5]). Since the stress depends on local intensity it will be greatest for an unscanned beam (M-mode and pulsed Doppler) at the *in situ* focus. It increases with increasing frequency following the ultrasonic attenuation dependence on frequency. As with the interface, the radiation stress gradient varies across the beam, being greatest on the axis and lower at the boundaries of the beam. For this reason, again, shear will be experienced by tissue at the boundary of the beam, being a maximum where the radial rate of change of intensity is greatest, and also be greatest at the focus where the beam is narrowest.

Pulsed vs. continuous waves

Radiation stress is experienced by tissue only during the passage of the pulse. For pulse-echo and pulsed Doppler modes its magnitude therefore depends on the pulse-average intensity and not on the time-average intensity. As each pulse passes through the tissue, it experiences a brief stress wave, which is carried with the pulse as it propagates. This can perhaps be likened to a peristaltic wave travelling along the pulse trajectory. Between pulses, no stress is applied to the tissue. For an interface, the radiation pressure is exerted only during the pulse period, the force being applied impulsively (like tapping a nail) rather than steadily (like pressing in a drawing pin or thumb tack). However, it should be emphasized that the forces involved, even during the pulse, are still very weak. Estimated values are given in Table 1.

Table 1 Calculated time-averaged and pulse-averaged radiation forces, pressures and gradients, caused by a 3-MHz pulse of temporal average intensity of 1 W/cm² and pulse average intensity 500 W/cm² (I_{SPPA}); beam area 10 mm²

	Totally absorbing interface	Tissue-like attenuating medium
Time-averaged force or gradient	65 µN	0.2 µN/mm
Time-averaged radiation pressure or gradient	6.5 Pa	0.02 Pa/mm
Pulse-averaged force or gradient	32.5 mN	0.1 mN/mm
Pulse-averaged radiation pressure or gradient	3.25 kPa	10 Pa/mm

For continuous wave ultrasound, as used in fetal heart monitors or ultrasonic physiotherapy, the tissue experiences a steady stress, rather than an intermittent one. However, since the highest intensities used in physiotherapy are about 100 times below the highest pulse-average intensities used in diagnostic systems, the stress experienced from absorption of sound in tissue during physiotherapy is similarly at least 100 times lower than that which may be achieved in a diagnostic pulse. The intensities delivered by fetal heart monitors are 100 times smaller still.

Other radiation forces

The forces discussed so far occur because of gradients in the energy density in the wave, for example at an acoustic interface or as a result of energy absorption by a homogeneous material. Other forces become effective if the medium is not homogeneous; it lies outside the scope of this review to discuss these forces, and for information on this topic, other reviews should be consulted[2]. In one interesting illustrative experiment[6] stasis and banding of erythrocytes was caused *in vivo*, in the circulation of a chick embryo, because of the forces acting on the blood cells in a standing wave field. Under these special conditions the energy density varies periodically, causing local aggregation of particles, such as cells, in the surrounding fluid. For the short pulse lengths used in diagnostic ultrasound, conditions tending to cause erythrocyte banding can occur only transiently near a strongly reflecting interface (bone or lung). For this reason the dramatic cell stasis illustrated by Dyson and colleagues[6] seems not to be relevant in judgements of diagnostic ultrasound safety, although transient stress adjacent to interfaces needs further study[7]. The greatest forces exerted by ultrasound on cells in suspension result from acoustic cavitation, and it is generally accepted that induced bubble oscillation, and the resulting shear forces induced adjacent to the bubble as a consequence, is the mechanism responsible for the hemolysis caused by ultrasound[8].

Finally a brief note should be added comparing the way heating, cavitation and radiation stress depend on other acoustic quantities, and consequently how bioeffects experiments may be interpreted. In a pulsed beam, bioeffects that are dependent on time-average intensity are interpreted as being of thermal origin, whilst those which depend on pulse amplitude are commonly interpreted as being due to cavitation. In pulsed beams radiation stress depends on pulse average intensity, and thus might well be a relevant alternative mechanism in any experiment showing pulse amplitude dependence. In such situations, care is needed for independent confirmation of the existence of cavitation activity before it is assumed to be the dominant bioeffects mechanism.

ACOUSTIC STREAMING

Having established that a small but finite internal stress field is always established within the body during the passage of ultrasound, the next question to address is what actual outcomes may result. For liquids, the outcome may be observed directly, as fluid motion along the direction of the beam. This overall liquid flow caused by the forward internal forces exerted within the fluid by the absorption of ultrasound is termed *acoustic streaming*, earlier known as 'quartz wind' when its origin was misinterpreted as being the transducer itself. It was first noted apparently by Faraday[1] in air above a vibrating plate, and has been the subject of a number of reviews[5, 9]. It is easy to imagine that the internal forward pressure gradient within the fluid would, indeed, tend to push it forward. As described above, the magnitude of the local forwardly directed force depends only on the local intensity and the attenuation. In a large enclosure, much larger than the beamwidth, fluid viscosity provides a retarding force that slows the fluid flow and limits the maximum velocity which may be reached in the beam. In addition, as the fluid space becomes comparable with the beamwidth, boundary frictional forces limit the maximum achievable streaming velocity.

Streaming in diagnostic exposures

For biomedical ultrasound beams it was long assumed that, whilst low-velocity acoustic streaming might be associated with continuous wave physiotherapy intensities, diagnostic ultrasound would not have the capacity to cause significant fluid movement under any conditions. However, Starritt and co-workers[10] demonstrated that the standard ultrasonic field conditions used by diagnostic scanners do, indeed, cause acoustic streaming in water (Figure 2). The greatest streaming velocity reported was 14 cm/s in a pulsed Doppler field from a commercial scanner at 3.5 MHz with free-field intensity [I_{SPTA}] of 4.0 W/cm². Of equal interest was the observation that streaming was generated in water by some imaging fields at the highest intensities, although the velocities were no more than 2 cm/s under these conditions.

It is clear from these studies[10] that continuous wave conditions are not necessary to sustain the driving force causing the stream, and that fluid movement can be generated as a result simply of a sequence of brief pulses traversing the fluid. This is true even if the time separation between

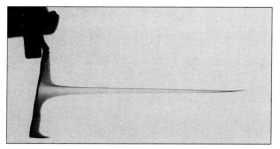

Figure 2 Streaming visualized in water by a pH indicator method. The streaming was caused by a pulsed Doppler beam. From reference 15 with permission from IOP Publishing Ltd.

pulses is as long as one imaging frame period, about 0.05 s. This implies that the passage of a single pulse through a liquid is sufficient to cause a relative displacement of the fluid in the beam with respect to the surrounding volume. Other important details given in this paper were that the streaming profile and the intensity profile were closely similar, and that the maximum velocity was reached at the focus. Furthermore, the time taken to establish the stream after switching on the beam was studied, and the few tenths of a second required is well within the dwell time (i.e. the duration that a single point tissue target receives ultrasound energy directly from the beam) used in clinical practice. Even for imaging, stable streams could be established within a few seconds. Acoustic non-linearity and shock formation were shown to be of considerable importance in increasing the streaming velocity. This is discussed further below.

Streaming in biological materials

Whilst the above study was valuable in revealing the capability of diagnostic beams to cause streaming, and hence cast some light on the underlying forces at play during the passage of diagnostic pulses, it was limited to investigating streaming in water. It is of considerable importance to ask what is likely to happen in other liquids, including those biological liquids relevant to scanning such as urine, amniotic fluid and blood. If the boundaries of the liquid volume are ignored for the present, the streaming velocity depends on the ratio of the attenuation to the viscosity. As is shown in Table 2, biological fluids are both more viscous and more absorbing than water. However, since the increase in absorption is proportionally greater

Table 2 Comparison of ultrasonic attenuation coefficient, α, at 1 MHz and relative viscosity, η, at room temperature. Streaming velocity depends on α/η. Data from reference 37, and P. K. Verma (personal communication)

Medium	Ultrasonic attenuation coefficient at 1 MHz, α (dB/cm)	Relative viscosity η
Water	0.0022	1
Amniotic fluid	0.005	1.1
Plasma	0.07	2.0
Whole blood	0.21	4.5

than the increase in viscosity, it might be expected that the streaming velocities achievable in biological fluids could be greater than those reached in water. Some studies using polythene solutions of different attenuation and viscosity have been carried out[11], and some studies with blood *in vitro* (F.R. Betheras, personal communication) suggest that this may be so.

One other circumstance when fluid movement has been observed has been during bioeffects experiments *in vitro*. For example, insonated rat embryos[12] were seen to move within the tube during exposure. Under the pulsed exposure conditions used, acoustic streaming would have been expected in the culture medium, and this is probably the explanation of the movement observed. Such movement of cells and organisms in experiments of this sort means that great care must be exercised in quantifying exposure, since the fluid contents of the experiment will be continually mixed by the acoustic stream. Whilst forces on organisms themselves also exist, these are insufficient to cause significant relative movement in free-field conditions at diagnostic levels, and only become dominant under the particular set of conditions which occur in a standing wave.

Streaming *in vivo*

Acoustic streaming has been noted by a number of clinical users of ultrasound, although their observations have not been well presented in the literature so far. *In vivo* streaming in a testicular abscess in an imaging field has been observed (H. B. Meire, personal communication). Fluid movement in a variety of fluid spaces *in vivo* has been studied as a potential diagnostic tool[13]. In one case streaming was observed in a post-hemorrhagic dilatation of the lateral ventricles of a premature infant, with the use of standard clinical pulsed Doppler equipment. Velocities as high as 18 cm/s have been recorded in blood *in vivo* (F.R. Betheras, personal communication). Fluid movement in breast cyst fluid caused by an ultrasound field has been observed and was suggested as a diagnostic technique for distinguishing fluid-filled from dense lesions[14].

Streaming in limited spaces

In most of these cases the estimated fluid velocities were relatively slow, of the order of 1 cm/s. One cause must be that these fluid movements were induced in confined spaces, and the size of the space containing the field is known to control the achievable speed. The importance of the size of the fluid volume has been studied experimentally for a diagnostic beam in water[15]. It was demonstrated that at the focus streaming velocities about 50% of the free-field velocity could be achieved within 5 mm of a transonic membrane in the beam. Neither a tube surrounding the beam about three times its width, nor a downstream membrane made any measurable change to the stream velocity. It may be concluded that fluid enclosed in spaces at least as small as 1 cm^3, and possibly smaller, should be induced to stream if exposed at the focus of pulsed Doppler beams at their highest intensities. No direct observations of streaming in obstetrics applications have been reported, but given the knowledge of acoustic streaming outlined above it can be stated with some confidence that fluid movement does occur in the main liquid spaces exposed to ultrasound – amniotic fluid and urine – during pulsed Doppler studies, and possibly during scanning. Elsewhere, in the fetal circulation, for example, the modifying effect on flow due to the acoustic forces described remain uncertain.

Non-linear propagation effects

It was noted above that the inherent non-linearity associated with the propagation of diagnostic pulses is of considerable importance in explaining the magnitude of streaming velocities achieved in diagnostic streams. A brief explanation will now be given; more detailed reviews of the importance of non-linear propagation in medical ultrasound are given elsewhere[16].

When a pulse of ultrasound travels away from a transducer, it does not retain its 'text-book' oscillatory form[17]. Typical alterations in waveform are shown in Figure 3. These changes occur because different parts of the pulse travel

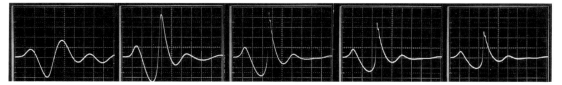

Figure 3   The development of pulse distortion as a diagnostic ultrasound pulse propagates through water

at different speeds. Specifically, the compressions in the pulse move faster than the rarefactions. Because it is physically impossible for the compression to overtake the rarefaction in front, after typically a few centimeters of travel an acoustic shock can form between a rarefaction and the compression behind it. (Surface waves on the sea undergo comparable alterations in shape as they approach the sea-shore, but in this case the wave crest overtakes the trough, forming a breaker). The acoustic shock so formed is an abrupt and sudden change in pressure where the shock thickness depends on the attenuation of the material; in water the shock can be as little as 10 nm thick.

Once the pulse has altered its form, its frequency content can no longer be described as a simple pulse spectrum centered around a specific frequency. Higher frequencies have been generated at harmonics of the fundamental. Rather than considering a pulse, it is easier to think of the alteration that occurs in a simple sinusoidal wave which ultimately forms a 'saw-tooth wave'. The spectrum of the sinusoid is at a single frequency. That of the saw-tooth is rich in harmonic content, whose amplitudes are proportional to 1/(harmonic number): for example, for a 1-MHz wave, the saw-tooth would contain 2 MHz at half the amplitude of the 1 MHz wave, 3 MHz at one-third the amplitude, and so on. As ultrasonic attenuation increases with increasing frequency, whether for water or body tissue, energy is absorbed more strongly from these shocked or saw-tooth waves than from the unmodified sine-wave. The local absorption is no longer simply that calculated from the material absorption coefficient, but can be considerably higher and is controlled by the ultrasonic character of the beam rather than the material properties of the propagation medium[18]. This rather odd situation applies

most strongly to water and weak aqueous solutions such as amniotic fluid, although it still applies to a lesser extent in soft tissue, and has been explored as a mechanism for enhanced tissue heating[19]. As the internal radiation stress (applied to the material) depends on the local attenuation, this too is increased when pulses are altered by non-linear waveform distortion and harmonic generation.

Starritt and co-workers[15] used a simple theoretical model to quantify the relative enhancement in the forward radiation stress gradient (the term radiation pressure gradient was used) when a saw-tooth rather than a sinusoidal wave was absorbed under a few conditions. With a 3-MHz wave, the radiation stress in water was enhanced by a factor of 180, that in amniotic fluid by 30 and in soft tissue by 4. Even so, the magnitude of the stress is still greatest in the most attenuating materials. Relative stress gradients for a few typical body components are shown in Figure 4. The application of improved models will enable new estimates to be made with greater confidence.

In an experimental study of acoustic streaming at diagnostic intensities in water, a six-fold enhancement in maximum streaming velocity was observed when comparing strongly shocked with quasi-linear conditions[10]. The time-averaged intensity was kept constant while the degree of non-linearity was altered by adjusting the pulse amplitude and timing. Other confirming measurements have subsequently been reported with the use of laser anemometry rather than thermal anemometry[11,20]. Furthermore, several recent theoretical analyses have confirmed and explored the phenomenon of shock-enhanced streaming[21-24].

In summary, the propagation of diagnostic ultrasound is strongly non-linear, most notably so in water and weak aqueous solutions, but also

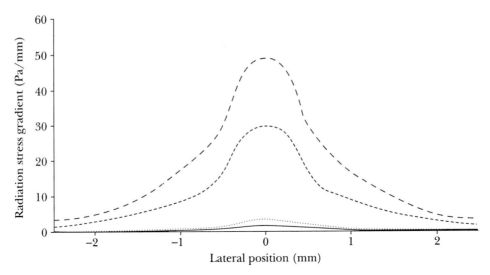

Figure 4 Radiation stress gradient profiles at the focus during the pulse of a fully shocked diagnostic beam in a number of biological materials. I_{SPPA} = 100 W/cm^2 Calculated from the measured intensity profile in water. Unbroken line, water; dotted line, amniotic fluid; short-dashed line, blood; long-dashed line, soft tissue

to some extent in the full range of soft tissues. The shocked waves generated within the body are more strongly absorbed than might be expected from simple linear calculations. For this reason the internal radiation stress on body components is enhanced to a degree which is dependent on the local non-linear distortion of the pulse. Enhanced streaming velocities have been demonstrated experimentally under such conditions and can now be predicted with some confidence.

WHAT HAPPENS IN TISSUES SUBJECT TO INTERNAL RADIATION STRESS?

Streaming

The internal stresses experienced as a result of the passage of diagnostic pulses are sufficient to displace liquids and cause streaming. The safety implications of this knowledge will now be explored. It would seem to be unlikely that the mere process of stirring amniotic fluid or urine would present any biophysical hazard. Similarly, the possible modification to blood flow in large vessels appears to be of little significance. The alteration of flow in smaller vessels must remain

speculative. Shear stress has been suggested as a potentiating factor in cell damage by heating[25]. It seems unlikely that present diagnostic devices can generate fluid streams capable of direct damage to cells in suspension from shear forces. At the boundary of a 2 mm diameter stream with a maximum velocity in water of 10 cm/s, shear is about 10 Pa, well below the threshold of 150 Pa for lysis of erythrocytes[26].

The possibility that ultrasound may enhance molecular diffusion through tissue, so-called phonophoresis, has been periodically studied, particularly with regard to alterations in transdermal drug transport by an ultrasonic field[27]. The evidence linking this effect to the internal forces outlined in this chapter is weak, however. Without exception, drug uptake enhanced by any physical agent can ultimately be related to increased skin perfusion, either because of mild heating or the presence of cavitation, and these seem to be the most likely mechanisms causing the enhancement of drug uptake by ultrasound. In principle the potential for altered transport of extracellular fluid exists, but explicit demonstration remains elusive. Diffusion at a cellular level also depends, for example, on osmotic pressure and surface tension, and evaluation of the disturbing effect of radiation forces is difficult. Perhaps the recent availability of magnetic resonance methods to explore diffusion *in vivo* may provide a method for experimental study in this area.

Physical alteration of soft tissue

The second subject for discussion concerns the outcome of these stresses on organized soft tissue. It is possible to consider two classes of response: that which manifests as a physical alteration of the tissue itself and a second class to do with sensory responses.

Predicting tissue displacement and possible direct damage is difficult, since the viscoelastic properties of tissue are complex and poorly investigated. Reported tensile strength of tissue is considerably higher than the stresses estimated above, that of even a weak tissue such as kidney parenchyma being 50 kPa[28]. However, comparisons are difficult, since it is probably the ultimate shear stress that is the critical quantity for assessing risk of mechanical damage, about which almost no objective data exist. Direct observations of the biophysical outcome of the stresses described are very few. It is certainly true that slight displacement of agar gel has been observed in continuous wave ultrasound[28], but unfortunately this study was at a much lower frequency, of 25 kHz. More useful observations of the direct effect of radiation stress have been made within the eye. Lizzi and co-workers[30], in work intended to cause retinal lesions, noted blanching of the choroid before the onset of thermal damage, which was interpreted as being caused by radiation pressure effects. This blanching was noted more readily when higher pulse amplitudes were used, and is therefore consistent with the view that the biophysical mechanism is radiation stress causing blood vessel compression. The pulse intensities (about 100 W/cm^2) were equivalent to those used diagnostically, but the pulse duration was longer: a minimum of 100 µs. The conclusion may be tentatively drawn that instantaneous radiation stresses achieved in diagnostic pulses are sufficient *if sustained* to cause compression ischemia. In other animal experiments visible motion of intravitreal substances, including dyes and vitreous membranes, have been reported[31,32].

As a general statement, the consensus is that adult soft tissues are not stressed to the point of physical damage by the forces exerted by diagnostic ultrasonic pulses. The contribution of radiation stress to ultrasonically generated lung hemorrhage remains uncertain.

Recently, evidence has been reported of hemorrhage within mouse fetal tissue, caused by ultrasound pulses, in the apparent absence of gas bodies[33]. In this study, Dalecki and colleagues used an experimental piezoelectric lithotripter (0.3 MHz) to deliver 200 pulses with amplitudes below 1 MPa, i.e. in the diagnostic range. The fetal tissues near developing bone or cartilaginous structures such as head, limbs and ribs showed evidence of hemorrhage. Adjacent soft tissues remained free of damage. Dalecki and co-workers speculated that, in the absence of other known mechanisms for damage, the hemorrhage could have resulted from relative motion between partially ossified bone and surrounding soft tissue. The bone may have been induced to move as a result of spatial variations in radiation force from local variations in the absorption coefficient. Further investigations are required to determine whether diagnostic level pulses can produce similar effects.

Streaming effects in obstetrics

Ultimately, the likelihood of cells being displaced with respect to their neighbor depends on the degree of tethering between them. Generally, all cells are in contact with a complex network of extracellular macromolecules called the extracellular matrix. Not only does this matrix act as the framework for cells, it also gives a lattice through which cells can migrate. Additionally, cells attach to one another by junctions, some of which (gap junctions) allow molecular communication between the cells. Of particular interest in the context of ultrasound safety is the cell structure of the embryo, in which the tissue strength depends very largely on cell-to-cell bonding, and the extracellular matrix has yet to develop to the point where it provides the structural strength it does in later fetal and adult life.

At the early embryonic stage, the soft extra-cellular material is primarily mucinous fluid and relatively poor in collagen, and most of the prospective fibrous tissues are still cellular[34]. Additionally, during the period of organogenesis (3.5–8 weeks' gestation in humans), cell migration and other complex cell–cell interactions occur, the coherence of which is essential to the viability and organization of the fetus. It is reasonable to speculate that this organization can tolerate only a finite mechanical internal strain without compromising subsequent development. The passage of a pulse-train through embryonic tissue could, in principle, exert sufficient radiation stress so that recovery from the resulting displacement would be unlikely. Whether such an effect could occur at diagnostic intensities is unclear. Nevertheless, this potential mechanism should be borne in mind whenever the outcome of bioeffect studies shows an effect that appears to depend neither on heating nor on cavitation. Any decisions to use diagnostic ultrasound during the first trimester should consider radiation stress as a potential bioeffect mechanism, and reduced exposures should be used.

Neurosensory responses

Several reports have appeared which implicate radiation stress as the biophysical mechanism responsible for neurosensory responses. It is possible to feel a pulsed ultrasound beam when it reaches the skin through a water bath, under appropriate conditions. In a study testing the origin of this sensation[35] it was demonstrated that the skin is sufficiently sensitive to detect radiation forces that are exerted by the absorption of beams with intensities of the order of $10–100 \text{ W/cm}^2$. The beams were either pulsed or modulated, i.e. turned on and off regularly at a frequency between 50 and 100 Hz. Thresholds for pulsed ultrasound were about ten times greater than those for a modulated beam, and increased substantially for pulses shorter than 1 ms. A minimum threshold for sensation for the modulated beam was about 0.4 mN. It was concluded that the sensation could be explained purely on the basis of radiation force. Ultrasound pulses of sufficient magnitude and

duration can alter cardiac function, and Dalecki and colleagues have recently examined the hypothesis of this resulting from radiation force[36]. During measurements on frog heart function two physiological responses to ultrasound were noted. These were premature ventricular contractions and a decrease in aortic blood pressure. Radiation force was confirmed as the most likely mechanism causing reduced blood pressure, but not for premature contractions. Estimated radiation force thresholds were about 3 mN for 5-ms pulses and 1 mN for 10-ms pulses. The studies were carried out at 1.2 and 3.7 MHz.

At sufficiently high pulse intensities, it is possible to stimulate a variety of other sensory receptors, which include heat and cold skin receptors, and pain receptors both at the skin and at depth[37]. For these studies, carried out over an extended range of frequencies, the threshold for the response most strongly correlated with particle displacement, rather than intensity or radiation pressure. In another study, Mihran and co-workers[38] interpreted alterations in the excitability of frog sciatic nerve *in vitro* following exposure to a single 0.5-ms pulse of ultrasound as being due to the associated radiation pressure transient.

Perhaps of most direct interest, however, are a number of reports which have demonstrated that the auditory nerve may be directly stimulated by ultrasound[39,40]; this includes one demonstrating that the pulse repetition frequency of a commercial pulsed Doppler system could be perceived by direct insonation via the foramen magnum[40]. The mechanism remains speculative, but one possibility is the direct effect of the varying stress field across the neural structures. The relevance of any of these studies to obstetric scanning remains speculative, but the possibility of some direct (but not necessarily hazardous) sensory stimulation of the fetus during ultrasound scanning cannot be ruled out.

ACKNOWLEDGEMENT

Useful commentary on an earlier draft of this paper by Dr Hazel Starritt is gratefully acknowledged.

References

1. Faraday, M. (1831). *Phil. Trans. R. Soc. (London)*, **121**, 229

2. Dunn, F. and Pond, J. B. (1978). Selected non-thermal mechanisms of interaction of ultrasound and biological media. In Fry, F.J. (ed.) *Ultrasound: Its Application in Medicine and Biology.* (New York: Elsevier)

3. Beissner, K. (1993). Radiation force and force balances. In Ziskin, M. C. and Lewin, P. A. (eds.) *Ultrasonic Exposimetry*, pp. 127–42. (Boca Raton: CRC Press)

4. Beyer, R. T. (1974). *Nonlinear Acoustics*, pp. 232–3. (US Department of the Navy)

5. Nyborg, W. L. (1953). Acoustic streaming due to attenuated plane waves. *J. Acoust. Soc. Am.*, **25**, 68–75

6. Dyson, M., Pond, J. B., Woodward, B. and Broadbent, J. (1974). The production of blood cell stasis and endothelial damage in blood vessels of chick embryos treated with ultrasound in a stationary wave field. *Ultrasound Med. Biol.*, **1**, 133–48

7. Duck, F. A. (1995). Radiation shear as a possible bioeffects mechanism. *Br. J. Radiol.*, **68**, 797 (abstr.)

8. Carstensen, E. L., Kelly, P., Church, C. C., Brayman, A. A., Child, S. Z., Raeman, C. H. and Schery, L. (1993). Lysis of erythrocytes by exposure to cw ultrasound. *Ultrasound Med. Biol.*, **19**, 147–65

9. Rooney, J. A. (1988). Other nonlinear acoustic phenomena. In Suslick, K. S. (ed.) *Ultrasound its Chemical, Physical, and Biological Effects.* (New York: VCH Publishers)

10. Starritt, H. C., Duck, F. A. and Humphrey, V. F. (1989). An experimental investigation of streaming in pulsed diagnostic ultrasound beams. *Ultrasound Med. Biol.*, **15**, 363–73

11. Mitome, H., Ishikawa, A., Takeda, H. and Kyoma, K. (1993). Effects of attenuation of ultrasound as a source of driving force of acoustic streaming. In Hobaek, H. (ed.) *Advances in Nonlinear Acoustics*, pp. 589–94. (Singapore: World Scientific)

12. Angles, J. M., Walsh, D. A., Li, K., Barnett, S. B. and Edwards, M. J. (1990). Effects of pulsed ultrasound and temperature on the development of rat embryos in culture. *Teratology*, **42**, 285–93

13. Betheras, F. R. (1990). Acoustic radiation force as a diagnostic modality. *Proceedings of the 20th Annual Conference of the Australian Society for Ultrasound in Medicine*, p. 69, Adelaide, September 1990

14. Nightingale, K. R., Kornguth, P. J., Walker, W. F., McDermott, B. A. and Trahey, E. G. (1995). A novel ultrasonic technique for differentiating cysts from solid lesions: preliminary results in the breast. *Ultrasound Med. Biol.*, **21**, 745–51

15. Starritt, H. C., Duck, F. A. and Humphrey, V. F. (1991). Forces acting in the direction of propagation in pulsed ultrasound fields. *Phys. Med. Biol.*, **36**, 1465–74

16. Muir, T. G. and Carstensen, E. L. (1980). Prediction of non-linear acoustic effects at biomedical frequencies and intensities. *Ultrasound Med. Biol.*, **6**, 345–57

17. Duck, F. A. and Starritt, H. C. (1984). Acoustic shock generation by ultrasonic imaging equipment. *Br. J. Radiol.*, **57**, 231–40

18. Dalecki, D., Carstensen, E. L., Parker, K. J. and Bacon, D. R. (1991). Absorption of finite amplitude focused ultrasound. *J. Acoust. Soc. Am.*, **89**, 2435–47

19. Swindell, W. (1985). A theoretical study of nonlinear effects with focused ultrasound in tissues: an 'acoustic Bragg peak'. *Ultrasound Med. Biol.*, **11**, 121–30

20. Duck, F. A., MacGregor, S. A. and Greenwell, D. (1993). Measurement of streaming velocities in medical ultrasonic beams using laser anemometry. In Hobaek, H. (ed.) *Advances in Nonlinear Acoustics*, pp. 607–12. (Singapore: World Scientific)

21. Mitome, H., Kozuka, T. and Tuzuiti, T. (1995). Effects of nonlinearity in development of acoustic streaming. *Jpn. J. Appl. Phys.*, **34**, 2584–9

22. Wu, J. and Du, G. (1993). Acoustic streaming generated by a focused Gaussian beam and finite amplitude tonebursts. *Ultrasound Med. Biol.*, **19**, 167–76

23. Kamakura, T., Matsuda, K., Kumamoto, Y. and Breazeale, M. A. (1995). Acoustic streaming induced in focused Gaussian beams. *J. Acoust. Soc. Am.*, **97**, 2740–6

24. Tjotta, S. and Tjotta, J. N. (1993). Acoustic streaming in ultrasound beams. In Hobaek, H. (ed.) *Advances in Nonlinear Acoustics*, pp. 601–6 (Singapore: World Scientific)

25. Dunn, F. (1985). Cellular inactivation by heat and shear. *Radiat. Environ. Biophys.*, **24**, 131–9

26. Leverett, L. B., Hellums, J. D., Alfrey, C. P. and Lynch, E. C. (1972). Red cell damage by shear stress. *Biophys. J.*, **12**, 257–73

27. Tachibana, K. and Tachibana, S. (1991). Transdermal delivery of insulin by ultrasonic vibration. *J. Pharm. Pharmacol.*, **43**, 270–1

28. Yamada, H. (1973). In Evans, F. G. (ed.) *Strength of Biological Materials*. (New York: Robert E. Krieger)

29. Dyer, H. J. and Nyborg, W. L. (1960). Ultrasonically induced movements in cells and cell models. *IRE Trans. Med. Elec.*, **ME-7**, 163–5

30. Lizzi, F. L., Coleman, D. J., Driller, J., Franzen, L. A. and Leopold, M. (1981). Effects of pulsed ultrasound on ocular tissue. *Ultrasound Med. Biol.*, **7**, 245–52

31. Coleman, D. J., Lizzi, F. L., Weininger, R. and Burt, W. (1970). Vitreous dispersion by ultrasound. *Ann. Ophthalmol.*, **2**, 389–96

32. Coleman, D. J., Lizzi, F. L., El-Mofty, A. A., Driller, J. and Franzen, L. (1980). Ultrasonically accelerated resorption of vitreous membranes. *Am. J. Ophthalmol.*, **89**, 490–9

33. Dalecki, D., Child, S. Z., Raeman, C. H., Penney, D. P., Mayer, R., Cox, C. and Carstensen, E. L. (1997). Thresholds for fetal haemorrhages produced by a piezoelectric lithotripter. *Ultrasound Med. Biol.*, **23**, 287–97

34. Willis, R. A. (1958). *The Borderland of Embryology and Pathology*, pp. 55–7. (London: Butterworth)

35. Dalecki, D., Child, S. Z., Raeman, C. H. and Carstensen, E. L. (1995). Tactile perception of ultrasound. *J. Acoust. Soc. Am.*, **97**, 3165–70

36. Dalecki, D., Raeman, C. R., Child, S. Z. and Carstensen, E. L. (1997). Effects of pulsed ultrasound on the frog heart: III. The radiation force mechanism. *Ultrasound Med. Biol.*, **23**, 275–85

37. Gavrilov, L. R. (1984). Use of focused ultrasound for stimulation of nerve structures. *Ultrasonics*, **22**, 132–8

38. Mihran, R. T., Barnes, F. S. and Wachtel, H. (1990). Temporally-specific modification of myelinated axon excitability *in vitro* following a single ultrasound pulse. *Ultrasound Med. Biol.*, **16**, 297–309

39. Tsirulnikov, E. M., Vartanyan, I. A., Gerunsi, G. V., Rosenblyum, A. S., Pudov, V. I. and Gavrilov, L. R. (1988). Use of amplitude-modulated focused ultrasound for diagnosis of hearing disorders. *Ultrasound Med. Biol.*, **14**, 277–85

40. Magee, T. R. and Davies, A. H. (1993). Auditory phenomena during transcranial Doppler insonation of the basilar artery. *J. Ultrasound Med.*, **12**, 747–50

Studies of ultrasound safety in humans: clinical benefit vs. risk

10

J. P. Newnham

SUMMARY

The safety of prenatal ultrasound in humans has never been addressed by a comprehensive, randomized controlled trial designed specifically to investigate the biological consequences of tissue insonation. However, data from controlled trials which were performed for other purposes, together with case–control studies and population cohorts, provide reasonable evidence that prenatal ultrasound scanning does not cause malformations or malignancy. Evidence from one randomized controlled trial of multiple prenatal scans suggests a small effect on birth weight which was not accompanied by any other deleterious effects, and was followed by catch-up growth during the first year of postnatal age. Several other studies have provided weak evidence for effects on subsequent speech and handedness, but our knowledge of the effects of ultrasound scanning on development of the central nervous system remains incomplete.

While reassurance can be gained from the current literature, the increasing use and intensity of ultrasound in the prenatal period demands our continuing investigation and vigilance.

INTRODUCTION

When Hippocrates preached the ideal of 'first do no harm', his comments would have been made in an environment of patients suffering from significant pathology. Today, we are faced with a new challenge which has arisen from the widespread availability of screening tests applied to people of whom most are entirely healthy. In this context, the chance of harm can easily exceed the chance of benefit. Most pregnancies now insonated for diagnostic purposes are entirely normal, rendering it imperative that we exclude any chance of harm from the exposure.

Since 1958 when diagnostic ultrasound was first applied to medicine[1], there have been numerous and extensive investigations of the safety of this clinical test. Studies have been performed on the biophysical consequences of tissue insonation, the effects on cells and whole animals, and the clinical outcome in humans. This chapter reviews the clinical and epidemiological studies as they relate to bioeffects in the human fetus.

RESEARCH METHODOLOGIES

The tools of the clinical research trade range from case reports based on anecdotal experience through to randomized controlled trials. Although each methodology has its strengths and weaknesses, the rigor and validity of evidence from each can be listed to form a hierarchy, as shown in Table 1[2].

The randomized controlled trial is accepted as the best method to assess the effectiveness of a test[3]. In this study design, subjects are allocated at random either to have the test (the intervention or treatment group) or not to have the test

Table 1 The hierarchy of evidence

Randomized controlled trials
Non-concurrent cohorts
Case–control studies
Historical control studies
Case series surveys
Case reports
Rumor

(the control group). Any differences between the groups in outcome can be attributed to the intervention. The effectiveness of diagnostic ultrasound has been subjected to a variety of randomized controlled trials and these are reviewed in Chapter 11. However, there has not been a randomized controlled trial performed with the specific intent of investigating safety. Plans for such a trial were developed in the UK[4] but were abandoned in the 1970s.

In the absence of data from controlled trials designed specifically to investigate bioeffects, studies of lesser rigor in design gain importance. Many of these have been based on case–control methodology. In these studies, subjects with a certain outcome are compared with an equal or greater number of other subjects who do not have the adverse outcome, but who share other characteristics such as age, gender or health attributes. These retrospective studies suffer from an inherent weakness in that not all characteristics will be controlled for, often resulting in systematic bias.

In the hierarchy of evidence, the randomized controlled trial reigns supreme as the ideal method of investigation. However, in the search for potential bioeffects, this technique may not identify effects which occur infrequently or first appear after data collection has concluded. If randomized controlled trials are to detect outcomes which are infrequent, the sample sizes need to be large. Ziskin and Petitti[5] have demonstrated that for a trial of ultrasound in pregnancy to investigate whether the rate of congenital anomalies were to be increased from a baseline of 5% to a new rate of 5.5%, a total 5200 subjects would need to be recruited for the finding to achieve statistical significance. Accordingly, the detection of infrequent and unexpected outcomes often relies on case reports and surveys, and the literature based on these methods needs to be monitored closely.

CONGENITAL MALFORMATIONS

Organogenesis in the human fetus occurs between days 24 and 55 following conception and during this time ultrasound examinations are often performed. Concerns that fetal develop-ment may be affected by environmental and therapeutic agents have been fuelled by widespread knowledge in the general community of several outstanding examples. Most prominent have been the links between thalidomide ingestion during the first trimester and subsequent limb defects in the child, diethylstilbestrol therapy given to women to prevent pregnancy loss and subsequent genital tract abnormalities and malignancy in the offspring, and rubella infection in the first trimester causing mental retardation, blindness and deafness.

At this time, there is general consensus based on reasonable evidence that ultrasound exposure does not cause congenital malformations. This evidence has come from regional malformation registers, specific studies and our understanding of the underlying principles.

Congenital malformation registries maintained during recent decades in which ultrasound exposure has increased do not report any change in the overall rates of malformation or of any specific defect which could be attributed to ultrasound use. The results of a national survey conducted in 1980 by the Environmental Health Directorate of Canada showed that no untoward effects were suspected after 1.2 million examinations in 340 000 pregnant women[6]. Reports such as this are highly reassuring, but cannot exclude small changes in the prevalence of abnormalities, in particular those in which the rates may alter for other reasons (such as prevention of neural tube defects by periconception folate therapy). Moreover, at the present time, evaluation of any effect of ultrasound exposure on congenital malformations would be confounded by the practice of interrupting pregnancies in which malformations have been diagnosed by ultrasound screening. Accordingly, the data from early studies have become invaluable in that diagnosis and termination of fetal abnormalities were less frequent then than occurs at present. These studies[7–11] are reviewed in Table 2 and indicate that congenital malformation rates were similar in pregnancies exposed to ultrasound when compared with matched controls.

Recently, Tikkanen and Heinonen[11] reported the results of a case–control study of all

Table 2 Clinical studies investigating prenatal diagnostic ultrasound exposure and congenital malformations

Reference	Exposure	Gestational age	Study design	Sample size	Findings
7	CW Doppler 20–30 mW/cm^2 6 MHz	10 weeks to term	case series	720	no increase in congenital malformations
8	PW imaging 10 mW/cm^2 2 MHz	throughout gestation	retrospective review	1114	no increase in congenital malformations
9	PW imaging I$_{SPTA}$ 4–28 mW/cm^2 2.25 or 3.5 MHz static and real-time6	throughout gestation	case–control	2428	no increase in congenital malformations
10	PW imaging	not stated	case–control matched for obstetric complications	425 exposed 381 controls	no increase in congenital malformations
11	PW imaging	first 16 weeks of pregnancy	case–control	406 cases 756 controls	congenital heart disease more frequent in ultrasound-exposed pregnancies; effect explained by greater frequency of threatened abortion

CW, continuous wave; PW, pulsed wave; I$_{SPTA}$, spatial peak temporal average intensity

101

cardiovascular malformations in Finland in 1982–83. The study investigated a role in the genesis of this malformation of maternal habits and exposures during pregnancy, including ultrasound examinations. Scans were performed in the first 16 weeks of pregnancy more frequently in the case group (28.3%) than among the control group (22.0%), although this difference did not achieve statistical significance. However, there was a significant increase in threatened abortion in the cases subsequently shown to have congenital heart disease, and when this association was accounted for in logistic regression analysis, it became clear that the possible link between ultrasound and congenital heart disease was not causal, but resulted from the performance of ultrasound in pregnancies complicated by threatened abortion. This study highlights the potential pitfalls in case–control studies and the need to account for confounding variables.

BIRTH WEIGHT

The most prominent and enduring feature in the scientific literature on potential bioeffects from ultrasound is a possible effect on birth weight. In small animal models, this endpoint has been noted in a proportion of the studies; these are reviewed in detail in Chapter 5. At this time, the literature describing research with laboratory animals remains inconclusive but it has provided the impetus for numerous clinical investigations.

In 1982, Moore and co-workers[12] reported in abstract form the results of a retrospective comparison of more than 2000 pregnancies, half of which had been exposed to diagnostic ultrasound. They observed a reduction in birth weight of 116 g in the exposed newborns, a difference which was statistically significant. The potential importance of this observation is diminished by the fact that the control group was not adequately matched and there was no account of the reason why the scan had been performed. It is entirely plausible that in such a retrospective comparison, the scanned group would contain a higher proportion of poorly grown fetuses, this being the clinical indication for the test. In addition, gestational age at birth was not controlled for and in a general clinical setting we would expect investigations of poor fetal growth to lead to obstetric intervention and an earlier age at birth. A subset of these data was subsequently reported by Stark and co-workers[10] who matched the exposed and unexposed groups for hospital of delivery and obstetric complications. In this analysis, no difference was observed in birth weight between the two groups.

Table 3 summarizes non-randomized clinical studies[10,12–17] investigating ultrasound exposure and size at birth.

Moore and co-workers[16] reported a retrospective comparison of exposed and unexposed pregnancies which had been delivered at Johns Hopkins Hospital in Baltimore during the calendar year 1981. Multivariate analyses were used in an attempt to account for the reason for the test. Exposure to more than one ultrasound scan, and first exposure during the third trimester, were both associated with a reduction in birth weight. However, the maternal and fetal risk factors that led to the performance of the scan appeared to be the major factors contributing to the birth weight difference.

The retrospective studies largely reported during the 1980s continued to suggest, but failed to prove, a link between ultrasound exposure and fetal growth. The inherent weakness in retrospective study designs, and the inability of statistical methodology completely to account for reasons that the scan was performed, left the question unanswered at the end of the decade. In more recent years, improvements in research methodology led to the publication of several randomized controlled trials. None of these trials was designed to investigate the safety of prenatal ultrasound, but the data nevertheless are invaluable. Some of the early trials were designed to test the hypothesis that releasing ultrasound data to clinicians would lead to improvements in pregnancy management. In these trials, there were similar scanning rates in the intervention and control groups, negating the opportunity to examine potential health effects[18,19].

Table 3 Non-randomized clinical studies investigating ultrasound exposure and size at birth

Reference	Exposure	Gestational age	Study design	Sample size	Findings
13	PW imaging 1–20 mW/cm² 2.25 MHz	14–20 weeks (mode 16) at time of amniocentesis	retrospective comparison of three cohorts	amniocentesis and ultrasound-exposed, 297 amniocentesis and ultrasound-unexposed, 661 neither amniocentesis nor ultrasound-exposed, 949	no differences in weight, length or head circumference at birth or at 1 year of age
12	PW imaging	not stated	comparison of two cohorts; controls not matched for obstetric indication for scan, gestational age at birth or time of exposure	exposed, 1061 unexposed, 1074	statistically significant reduction in birth weight of exposed fetuses (116 g)
14	PW imaging	throughout gestation	comparison of two physicians' practices: one using ultrasound, the other not	ultrasound-exposed, 315 non-exposed, 270	no difference in birth weight
10	PW imaging	not stated	case–control subset of reference 12 study; controlled for obstetric complications and hospital of delivery	exposed, 425 unexposed, 381	no difference in birth weight
15	PW imaging static and real time 4–28 mW/cm² 2.25 or 3.5 MHz	throughout gestation; 55% in second trimester	case–control: matched sibling pairs of same sex	149 pairs	no differences in weight, length or head circumference at birth, or height and weight at 6 years of age
16	PW imaging	throughout gestation	comparison of two patient groups	exposed, 1598 non-exposed, 944	lower birth weight in exposed fetuses; could not be separated from reason why scan was performed
17	PW imaging	throughout gestation	case–control, using health insurance data	exposed, 940 controls, 3749	no increase in low birth weight in exposed group

PW, pulsed wave

Two randomized controlled trials performed in Europe[20,21] compared protocols of one or two scans vs. a policy of no routine scans in the control group. In each of these studies, the primary aim was to reduce the rate of induction of labor for 'post-term' by improving the accuracy of dating. Mean birth weight was greater in the scanned groups and in one study the difference achieved statistical significance[21]. It was speculated that the ultrasound examinations encouraged women to reduce smoking, resulting in an improvement in birth weight.

In a large trial performed in Finland, commonly known as 'The Helsinki Ultrasound Trial', 9310 women were allocated at random to a policy of routine screening at 16–20 weeks' gestation or to a policy of selected screening only[22]. In these two groups, the mean number of ultrasound scans was 2.1 and 1.8, respectively. There was no significant difference in birth weight between the two groups. More recently, Ewigman and colleagues[23] reported the results of a trial of more than 15 000 women in which a random half were allocated to a policy of a scan at 15–22 weeks' gestation, with a further scan at 31–35 weeks, or to a control group which underwent scans for medical reasons only. This trial was performed in North America and is commonly known as 'The RADIUS Study'. The mean number of scans in these two groups was 2.2 and 0.6, respectively. Birth weight distributions in the two groups were almost identical.

Other studies[24–28] using randomized controlled trials to determine an association between prenatal ultrasound and weight at birth are summarized in Table 4. Together, the results of these randomized controlled trials provide compelling evidence that one or two imaging scans in pregnancy do not affect the weight of the infant at birth.

The same assurances cannot be given for multiple scans. There has been only one report of a randomized controlled trial in which multiple scans were studied and in this trial a possible effect on growth was observed. Newnham and co-workers[29] allocated at random 1415 women with single pregnancies at 16–20 weeks' gestation to a protocol of ultrasound imaging and Doppler flow studies at 18, 24, 28, 34 and 38 weeks' gestation (the intensive group) and 1419 women to receive a single scan at 18 weeks' gestation with further scans as clinically indicated (the regular group). The study was performed at the tertiary level perinatal center in Western Australia between 1989 and 1992. Each imaging study involved fetal biometry and assessment of amniotic fluid volume and placental site. The Doppler flow studies of the flow velocity waveforms from umbilical and uteroplacental arteries were performed with standalone continuous wave equipment.

Mean birth weight in the intensive group was 25 g less than in the regular group, a difference that did not achieve statistical significance. However, the proportion of live born infants with birth weight less than the 10th centile, and less than the 3rd centile, were greater in the intensive group (relative risk 1.35, 95% confidence interval 1.09–1.67, $p = 0.006$; and 1.65, 1.09–2.49, $p = 0.02$, respectively). This difference between the two groups in the lower birth weight centiles could not be explained by differential clustering of maternal characteristics or smoking practices, gestational ages at birth, or obstetric intervention[30]. No other differences were observed between the two groups. In particular, there were similar pregnancy outcomes as measured by duration of neonatal stay, requirements for resuscitation and events in the neonatal nursery. Comparison between the two groups of measurements made on the second or third day of life revealed a trend for those in the intensive ultrasound group to be shorter, and not to have a relative reduction in soft tissue growth[31]. While analysis of neonatal biometry was not conclusive, the observations suggested that if multiple scans do indeed restrict fetal growth, the mechanism is more likely to be an effect on bone growth than a reduction in nutrient supply from the placenta. When examined at 1 year of age, the children from the two arms of the trial were of similar weight[32]. Moreover, statistically significant catch-up growth had occurred in those who had been in the intensive ultrasound group. This observation provides further evidence that the weight difference observed at birth had been real, and that the effect on growth was transient and

Table 4 Randomized controlled trials of prenatal ultrasound and weight at birth

References	Intervention	Controls	Primary hypothesis	Sample size intervention: control	Findings
20	imaging at 19 and 32 weeks' gestation	no scan	reduction in induction for post-term pregnancy	510 : 499	mean birth weight 25 g higher in screened group (not significant)
21	single dating scan at 15 weeks (BPD measurement)	no scan for dating	(1) reduction in induction for post-term pregnancy (2) increased birth weight and gestational age of twins	2389 : 2412	mean birth weight 42 g higher in screened group (significant)
22	routine scan at 16–20 weeks (mean no. of scans = 2.1)	selective scans at 16–20 weeks (mean no. of scans = 1.8)	effects on medical services, obstetric procedures and fetal outcomes	4691 : 4619	mean birth weight 13 g higher in screened group (not significant)
24	CW Doppler scanning of umbilical artery	computerized fetal heart rate monitoring	reduction in time for fetal assessment	438 : 459	mean birth weight 4 g higher in controls (not significant)
25	routine CW Doppler studies up to monthly	standard care with no Doppler studies	effects on rate of antenatal hospital admission	1246 : 1229	no difference in proportions with birth weight < 10th centile
26	pulsed Doppler scanning of umbilical artery	fetal heat rate monitoring	Doppler better than FHR monitoring for fetuses with growth restriction	214 : 212	mean birth weight 63 g higher in intervention group (not significant)
23	routine scan at 15–22 weeks + another at 31–35 weeks (mean 2.2)	scans for medical indications only (mean 0.6)	effects on adverse perinatal outcomes (perinatal death or morbidity)	7812 : 7718	mean birth weight 4 g higher in screened group (not significant)
27	CW Doppler in 80% of cases	CW Doppler in only 3.9% of cases	Doppler in all low-risk primagravid women will lower obstetric intervention and neonatal morbidity	1015 : 1001	mean birth weight 27 g higher in controls (not significant)
28	CW Doppler	no access to Doppler	effect of introducing Doppler studies on obstetric outcome	1114 : 1175	mean birth weight 12 g higher in intervention group (not significant)
29	routine imaging scan and CW Doppler at 18, 24, 28, 34 and 38 weeks	single imaging at 18 weeks	reductions in neonatal hospital stay and rate of preterm birth	1415 : 1419	significant increase in birth weight < 10th centile in scanned group

BPD, biparietal diameter; CW, continuous wave; FHR, fetal heart rate apparently harmless. The children in this Western Australian trial remain under close observation and their ongoing growth and development will continue to provide invaluable data on the consequences of prenatal ultrasound exposure.

The Western Australian study provides the only data available from a randomized controlled trial in humans that can address the question of whether multiple scans affect fetal growth. However, a link between multiple ultrasound exposures and prenatal growth has not been proven. It was not the purpose of this trial to investigate the safety of ultrasound, but rather to test whether a protocol of multiple scans would lead to improvements in outcome[30]. Accordingly, an effect on birth weight was not a prior hypothesis. As such, the trial has not proved that multiple scans affect prenatal growth, but has provided evidence to support such a hypothesis. The intent and design of a trial are vital characteristics which must be considered when deciding whether a trial has proved a hypothesis, or has simply provided evidence to generate a hypothesis. A definitive trial is now required to address the question of whether multiple scans affect fetal growth. Could such a trial be performed? The results of the Western Australian study have shown that multiple scans do not result in measurable morbidity for the pregnancy or newborn and that any effect on growth appears to be harmless. However, to examine the hypothesis ideally would require the results of the scans to be blinded and the women in the control group to attend for the test but the ultrasound equipment not to be activated. Approval for such a trial might be difficult to obtain.

SENSORY AND NEUROLOGICAL DEVELOPMENT

There have been no studies designed with the specific intent to investigate the effects of prenatal ultrasound on sensory and neurological development in childhood. However, various tests have been performed on children who had been exposed to diagnostic ultrasound before birth in studies that had been performed to investigate hypotheses relevant to obstetric management. These studies are reviewed in Table 5.

One of the earliest investigations of the safety of prenatal ultrasound involved retrospective follow-up of infants from the Amniocentesis Registry of the US National Institute of Child Health and Human Development[13]. A group of 297 infants of women who had received both amniocentesis and ultrasound were compared with a group of 661 infants of women who had amniocentesis but no ultrasound and with 949 infants who had been exposed to neither amniocentesis nor ultrasound. Neurological findings at birth were similar in the three groups, apart from two signs – the grasp reflex and the tonic neck reflex – which were more frequently abnormal in the amniocentesis-with-ultrasound group than in the controls. The investigators noted that this finding may have resulted from a greater proportion of infants in the amniocentesis-with-ultrasound group being sick for other reasons; by the time of discharge from hospital, there were no differences between the three groups. Evaluation at 1 year of age included a Denver Developmental Scoring evaluation and history of hearing disorder and infections; infants in the three groups were again found to be similar.

Perhaps the most highly cited clinical evaluation of ultrasound safety during the 1980s was the retrospective case–control study reported by Stark and co-workers[10]. A total of 425 children exposed to prenatal ultrasound at three Denver hospitals between 1968 and 1972 were matched with 381 control children. Each child was examined at birth and again at 7–12 years of age. Newborn examinations involved assessment for anomalies and growth, as described earlier in this chapter. At 7–12 years of age there were no significant or consistent differences between the two groups in Wechsler Intelligence Scale for Children verbal and performance intelligence quotient scores, reading scores or Gray Oral total passage scores. Other tests that showed similar findings in the two groups included evaluation of the cranial nerves, co-ordination and reflexes. Hearing and visual systems were also tested. These tests showed no differences

Table 5 Studies of prenatal ultrasound and neurological development of the child

Reference	Exposure	Gestational age	Study design	Sample size	Findings
13	PW imaging 1–20 mW/cm^2 2.25 MHz	14–20 weeks (mode 16) at time of amniocentesis	retrospective comparison of three cohorts	amniocentesis and ultrasound exposed, 297 amniocentesis and ultrasound unexposed, 661 neither amniocentesis nor ultrasound, 949	transient neurological differences at birth in ultrasound exposed no neurological differences at 1 year of age
10	PW imaging number of scans not known	not stated	case–control	exposed, 425 unexposed, 381	no differences at 7–12 years of age in hearing, visual acuity or intellectual ability, but a suggestion of increased dyslexia
33	PW imaging	19 and 32 weeks	two randomized controlled trial cohorts	exposed, 1015 unexposed, 996	no differences at 8–9 years of age in school performance or rates of dyslexia
34	PW imaging (as above)	19 and 32 weeks (as above)	further studies of the two randomized controlled trial cohorts (as above)	exposed, 1115 unexposed, 1046	significant increase in non-right-handedness in screened children at 8–9 years of age no difference in allergies
36	not stated	not stated	case–control	72 cases each matched to two controls	delayed speech at 5 years of age more frequent in the ultrasound-exposed group

PW, pulsed wave

between the two groups in hearing acuity thresholds in the frequency range of 500–4000 Hz and no differences in nerve deafness as measured by the Wepman Auditory Discrimination Test. Visual acuity and color perception were similar in the exposed and unexposed groups. However, there were more children with dyslexia in the exposed group in each of the three hospitals. The authors performed χ^2 tests for each hospital group and noted that within each group statistical significance was not achieved. If the children from each group within the three hospitals are combined and the effect of ultrasound exposure tested by logistic regression analysis, the difference in dyslexia rates between the exposed and unexposed groups is statistically significant (odds ratio 1.39; 95% confidence interval 1.08–1.80; $p = 0.012$). This analysis cannot account for the obvious confounding effects of racial and cultural differences in the various populations attending each of the three hospitals. Again, the pitfalls inherent in any case–control study complicate our interpretation of this report. Indeed, the authors stated that the matching procedure tended to produce controls with fewer and less serious obstetric complications. It is of further concern that the ascertainment rate of cases and controls at 7–12 years of age was only 27%.

In 1992, the results were reported of examinations at 8–9 years of age of 2011 children who had participated in two prenatal ultrasound trials in Norway[33]. Women had been allocated at random to be offered a scan at 19 weeks and another at 32 weeks of pregnancy, or to a control group in which ultrasound examinations were not offered as a routine, although 19% received at least one scan. Analyses were conducted on an 'intention to treat' basis. The teachers of these children in primary school were asked to assess reading achievement, spelling and arithmetic, and to complete a measure of dyslexia. There were no differences between the screened and unscreened groups in any index of school performance. In view of the findings reported by Stark and colleagues[10] which had suggested a possible effect of ultrasound exposure on the prevalence of dyslexia, a subsample of 32% of the children was selected for specific

tests of dyslexia at 9–10 years of age. In this validation study, there were also no differences between the two groups in the rate of dyslexia.

In a subsequent report, Salvesen and colleagues[34] further explored the possible effect of ultrasound exposure on neuronal development. Since ultrasound screening often coincides with the stage in fetal development when neurons migrate towards their final destination in the brain, the prevalence of right-handedness (laterality) may be used as a marker of random damage to the cerebral hemispheres. The cohort of children from the two randomized controlled trials performed in Norway was again used. Information employed in the analysis was primarily obtained by questionnaires completed by the parents and from data collected in child health centers. The dominant hand was determined by the responses to ten specific questions answered by the mother. It was found that the prevalence of non-right-handedness was higher in children who had been exposed to prenatal ultrasound than among control children (odds ratio 1.32; 95% confidence interval 1.02–1.71). The authors acknowledged that the significant finding with handedness may have resulted from chance. This question had been one of six initial hypotheses and the apparent significance may have resulted from multiple analyses. Moreover, it remains possible that response rates of the mothers may have differed amongst those who were concerned that their child was left-handed, and that different ages of testing may have produced bias because the degree of handedness is known to change with age[35]. Appropriately, it has been concluded that children from other randomized controlled trials of prenatal ultrasound exposure need to be evaluated for handedness.

Speech is a developmentally defined symptom complex, delay of which may have numerous causal factors. In a study which addressed speech development, Campbell and co-workers[36] reported the results of a retrospective case–control study centered on 72 Canadian children who had been identified by speech–language pathologists to have delayed speech. It was specified that this classification required the delay in speech to be of unknown origin. The children were, on average, 5 years of age. Each case was matched with two controls selected for gender, date of birth, sibling birth order and associated health problems that were based on speech and hearing. The control children were similar to the cases in terms of gestational age and weight at birth. Children with delayed speech had a higher rate of prenatal ultrasound exposure than did the controls (odds ratio 2.8; 95% confidence interval 1.5–5.3, $p = 0.001$). It was concluded that a child with delayed speech is about twice as likely as a child without delayed speech to have been exposed to prenatal ultrasound. However, caution must be exercised in interpretation of this study. Of greatest concern is the fact this case–control study failed to match obstetric problems and no reasons were given for the performance of each scan[37]. In the presence of such a limitation in study design, it remains likely that the ultrasound scan was nothing more than a surrogate for the medical and obstetric complications which led to the test being performed. This study, and subsequent criticisms of its design, again highlight the limited ability of case–control studies to describe causation. The findings of impaired speech development were also not supported in a subsequent epidemiological study[38]. Nevertheless, the Canadian case–control study reporting delayed speech in children who had been exposed to prenatal ultrasound has placed the question of speech development firmly on the agenda of research priorities in this field.

MALIGNANCY

Two British case–control studies published together in 1984 compared the prenatal ultrasound histories of children with malignancy with those of matched controls[39,40]. The numbers of cases in these two studies were 1731 and 555, respectively. Exposure to prenatal ultrasound did not differ between the children who had cancer and the controls, apart from a small increase in cases exposed during the earlier years of ultrasound, a finding thought to reflect the selective application of scans to abnormal pregnancies at that time[39]. These studies have provided evidence that exposure of the fetus to ultrasound is not carcinogenic, although it must be appreciated that these studies were performed at a time when ultrasound dosages were less and the application more selective than often occurs in current clinical practice. As an example, the proportions of children in the entire obstetric population who had received ultrasound exposure before birth in these two studies were 6 and 26%, respectively, as compared with almost universal use of prenatal ultrasound in the current environment.

Since these landmark publications, a variety of other studies have provided further evidence that prenatal ultrasound is not carcinogenic[41,42]. The most recent of these was a population-based case–control study of 642 childhood cancer cases in Shanghai, China[43]. Prenatal ultrasound exposure was not associated with an increased risk of childhood cancer, but a strong association between fetal diagnostic X-rays and subsequent malignancy was again confirmed. Overall, prenatal X-ray use was followed by an 80% increased risk of childhood cancer.

DISCUSSION

At this time, an adverse effect of prenatal ultrasound exposure in humans has not been demonstrated with certainty, i.e. none has been independently verified. However, it is equally true that absolute safety has not been proven.

Most evidence for the safety of prenatal insonation in humans has come from a small number of case–control studies and follow-up of children from a few randomized controlled trials. In these studies, the scanning mostly involved only one or two examinations throughout the pregnancy, and used imaging equipment typical of clinical practice in the late 1970s and early 1980s. These studies provide reasonable evidence that scans of this type and frequency do not cause congenital malformations, do not affect birth weight and do not predispose the child to subsequent malignancy. One case–control study found weak evidence for an increased rate of dyslexia at 7–12 years of age[10], but a more extensive study of children at 8–9 years of age from a controlled trial has since provided stronger evidence that the prevalence of dyslexia is not increased by prenatal scanning[33]. One study reported an association between delay in speech development and prenatal insonation[36]; however, the design of this study was inadequate for a firm conclusion to be reached. Hearing has been addressed in one case–control study, and although it was concluded that prenatal scanning did not affect auditory development, the range of testing was restricted to 500–4000 Hz[10]. There has been no study of the effect of prenatal ultrasound on subsequent hearing in the higher frequency ranges. Evaluation of an effect on vision has also been limited.

It is surprising, and not to our collective credit, that a biophysical intervention used for diagnostic purposes is being applied to almost all unborn children in the developed world, yet its safety has never been investigated specifically in a controlled trial. This chapter has reviewed the evidence of safety which must be garnered from studies of lesser design and strength, the importance of which reflects the absence of more appropriate data. In the past, the principal issue was the safety of imaging scans at 16–20 weeks' gestation when most anatomy and dating scans were performed, and at approximately 32 weeks' gestation when most growth assessments were made. Today, many fetuses are exposed to ultrasound at a variety of other times, and with much greater intensities. A single case may now include follicle scanning prior to conception, transvaginal imaging and Doppler studies in the embryo stage, imaging scans as guidance for needle insertion procedures, several imaging and biometric scans in the second and third trimesters, electronic fetal heart rate monitoring based on continuous or pulsed wave Doppler during the third trimester, pulsed and color Doppler scanning of fetal and uterine perfusion and continuous insonation for up to 18 h or more by electronic fetal heart rate monitoring in labor. The safety and potential bioeffects of ultrasound exposure in such cases are not addressed by the data which currently exist in the literature. There has been a single randomized controlled trial in which multiple scans and Doppler studies were compared with a single imaging scan[29]. No effect on pregnancy outcome or neonatal morbidity was observed, but there was a significant increase in newborns in the lower birth weight centiles. Evidence of such strength should be seen as strong support for the initiation of a randomized controlled trial designed specifically to investigate the safety of multiple exposures to prenatal ultrasound.

The potential for untoward effects from widespread use of prenatal ultrasound must be weighed against the benefits which result from use of this technology. One outstanding advantage has been the ability of this diagnostic test to replace the use of X-rays. Radiographs were previously used to diagnose multiple pregnancies, to confirm the presentation and to assess the pelvic size and shape. For many children, the avoidance of X-rays during pregnancy has undoubtedly lessened their risk of malignancy.

This chapter has dealt exclusively with the potential health effects associated with prenatal exposure to diagnostic ultrasound. The issue of safety of prenatal ultrasound must also include the consequences of false-positive and false-negative findings. As will be reviewed in the following chapter, studies have reported considerable variance in the diagnostic accuracy of ultrasound tests[23,44], which for anatomy scanning at 18 weeks' gestation ranges from sensitivities of 16 to 84%. The factors making the greatest contributions to this variance are the skill and training of the operator and the quality of the equipment. While there is no place for complacency with regard to the potential for ultrasound-induced adverse effects, the evidence from clinical studies indicates that at this time the greatest danger faced by women and children from prenatal ultrasound may result from the consequences of diagnostic inaccuracy, rather than from the insonation itself.

References

1. Donald, I., MacVicar, J. and Brown, T. D. (1958). Investigation of abdominal masses by pulsed ultrasound. *Lancet*, **1**, 1188–95

2. Newnham, J. P. and Evans, S. F. (1995). Clinical evaluation of ultrasound technology. *Ultrasound Q.*, **13**, 103–10

3. Chalmers, I. (1989). Evaluating the effects of care during pregnancy and childbirth. In Chalmers, I., Enkin, M. and Keirse, M. J. N. C. (eds.) *Effective Care in Pregnancy and Childbirth*, pp. 3–38. (Oxford: Oxford University Press)

4. Mole, R. (1986). Possible hazards of imaging and Doppler ultrasound in obstetrics. *Birth*, **13**, 29–37

5. Ziskin, M. C. and Petitti, D. B. (1988). Epidemiology of human exposure to ultrasound: a critical review. *Ultrasound Med. Biol.*, **14**, 91–6

6. Environmental Health Directorate (1981). *Safety Code 23. Guidelines for the Safe Use of Ultrasound*, Part I. *Medical and Paramedical Applications*. Report 8-EHD-59. (Ottawa, Canada: Environmental Health Directorate, Health Protection Branch)

7. Bernstine, R. L. (1969). Safety studies with ultrasonic Doppler technique: a clinical follow-up of patients and tissue culture study. *Obstet. Gynecol.*, **34**, 707–9

8. Hellman, L. M., Duffus, G. M., Donald, I. and Sunden, B. (1970). Safety of diagnostic ultrasound in obstetrics. *Lancet*, **1**, 1133–5

9. Lyons, E. A. (1986). Human epidemiology studies. In Kossoff, G. and Barnett, S. B. (eds.) *1st WFUMB Symposium on Safety and Standardisation of Ultrasound in Obstetrics. Ultrasound Med. Biol.*, **12**, 689–91

10. Stark, C. R., Orleans, M., Haverkamp, A. D. and Murphy, J. (1984). Short and long-term risks after exposure to diagnostic ultrasound *in utero*. *Obstet. Gynecol.*, **63**, 194–200

11. Tikkanen, J. and Heinonen, O. P. (1992). Congenital heart disease in the offspring and maternal habits and home exposures during pregnancy. *Teratology*, **46**, 447–54

12. Moore, R. M., Barrick, M. K. and Hamilton, P. M. (1982). Ultrasound exposure during gestation and birthweight. Presented at the *15th Annual Meeting of the Society for Epidemiologic Research*, June, Cincinnati

13. Scheidt, P. D., Stanley, F. and Bryla, D. A. (1978). One-year follow-up of infants exposed to ultrasound *in utero*. *Am. J. Obstet. Gynecol.*, **131**, 743–8

14. Smith, C. B. (1984). Birthweights of fetuses exposed to diagnostic ultrasound. *J. Ultrasound Med.*, **3**, 395–6

15. Lyons, E. A., Dyke, C., Toms, M. and Cheang, M. (1988). *In utero* exposure to diagnostic ultrasound: a 6 year follow-up. *Radiology*, **166**, 687–90

16. Moore, R. M., Diamond, E. L. and Cavalieri, R. L. (1988). The relationship of birthweight and intrauterine diagnostic ultrasound exposure. *Obstet. Gynecol.*, **71**, 513–17

17. Grisso, J. A., Strom, B. L., Cosmatos, I., Tolosa, J., Main, D. and Carson, J. (1994). Diagnostic ultrasound in pregnancy and low birthweight. *Am. J. Perinatol.*, **11**, 297–301

18. Bennett, M. J., Little, G., Dewhurst, J. and Chamberlain, G. (1982). Predictive value of ultrasound measurement in early pregnancy: a randomised controlled trial. *Br. J. Obstet. Gynaecol.*, **89**, 338–41

19. Nielson, J. P., Munjanja, S. P. and Whitfield, C. R. (1984). Screening for small for dates fetuses: a controlled trial. *Br. Med. J.*, **289**, 1179–82

20. Bakketeig, L. S., Eik-Nes, S. H., Jacobsen, G., Ulstein, M. K., Brodtkorb, C. J., Balstad, P., Erikensen, B. C. and Jorgensen, N. P. (1984). Randomised controlled trial of ultrasonographic screening in pregnancy. *Lancet*, **2**, 207–11

21. Waldenstrom, U., Axelsson, O., Nilsson, S., Eklund, G., Fall, O., Linderberg, S. and Sjodin, Y. (1988). Effects of routine one-stage ultrasound screening in pregnancy: a randomised controlled trial. *Lancet*, **2**, 585–8

22. Saari-Kemppainen, A., Karjalainen, O., Ylöstalo, P. and Heinonen, O. P. (1990). Ultrasound screening and perinatal mortality: controlled trial of systematic one-stage screening in pregnancy. The Helsinki Ultrasound Trial. *Lancet*, **336**, 387–91

23. Ewigman, B. G., Crane, J. P., Frigoletto, F. D., LeFevre, M. L., Bain, R. P., McNeillis, D. and The RADIUS Study Group (1993). A randomised trial of prenatal ultrasound screening in a low risk population: impact on perinatal medicine. *N. Engl. J. Med.*, **329**, 821–7

24. Hofmeyr, G. J., Pattinson, R., Buckley, D., Jennings, J. and Redman, C. W. G. (1991). Umbilical artery resistance index as a screening test for fetal well-being. II: Randomised feasibility study. *Obstet. Gynecol.*, **78**, 359–62

25. Davies, J. A., Gallivan, S. and Spencer, J. A. D. (1992). Randomised controlled trial of Doppler ultrasound screening of placental perfusion during pregnancy. *Lancet*, **340**, 1299–303

26. Almstrom, H., Axelsson, O., Cnattingius, S., Ekman, G., Maesel, A., Ulmsten, U., Arstrom, K.

and Marsal, K. (1992). Comparison of umbilical-artery velocimetry and cardiotocography for surveillance of small-for-gestational-age fetuses. *Lancet,* **340**, 936–40

27. Mason, G. C., Lilford, R. J., Porter, J., Nelson, E. and Tyrell, S. (1993). Randomised comparison of routine versus highly selective use of Doppler ultrasound in low risk pregnancies. *Br. J. Obstet. Gynaecol.,* **100**, 130–3

28. Johnstone, F. D., Prescott, R., Hoskins, P., Greer, I. A., McGlew, T. and Compton, M. (1993). The effect of introduction of umbilical Doppler recordings to obstetric practice. *Br. J. Obstet. Gynaecol.,* **100**, 733–41

29. Newnham, J. P., Evans, S. F., Michael, C. A., Stanley, F. J. and Landau, L. I. (1993). Effects of frequent ultrasound during pregnancy: a randomised controlled trial. *Lancet,* **342**, 887–91

30. Newnham, J. P., Evans, S. F., Michael, C. A., Stanley, F. J. and Landau, L. I. (1993). Reply to letters to the editor: Effects of frequent ultrasound during pregnancy. *Lancet,* **342**, 1359–61

31. Evans, S., Newnham, J., MacDonald, W. and Hall, C. (1996). Characterisation of the possible effect on birthweight following frequent prenatal ultrasound examination. *Early Hum. Dev.,* **45**, 203–14

32. MacDonald, W., Newnham, J., Gurrin, L. and Evans, S. (1996). Effect of frequent prenatal ultrasound on birthweight: follow-up at one year of age. *Lancet,* **348**, 482

33. Salvesen, K. A., Bakketeig, L. S., Eik-Nes, S. H., Undheim, J. O. and Okland, O. (1992). Routine ultrasonography *in utero* and school performance at age 8–9 years. *Lancet,* **339**, 85–9

34. Salvesen, K. A., Vatten, L. J., Eik-Nes, S. H., Hugdahl, K. and Bakketeig, L. S. (1993). Routine ultrasonography *in utero* and subsequent handedness and neurological development. *Br. Med. J.,* **307**, 159–64

35. McManus, I. C. (1993). Ultrasonography and handedness (letter). *Br. Med. J.,* **307**, 563–4

36. Campbell, J. D., Elford, R. W. and Brant, R. F. (1993). Case–control study of prenatal ultrasonography exposure in children with delayed speech. *Can. Med. Assoc. J.,* **149**, 1435–40

37. Dyke, C. (1994). Studying delayed speech (letter). *Can. Med. Assoc. J.,* **150**, 647–8

38. Salvesen, K. A., Vatten, L. J., Bakketeig, L. S. and Eik-Nes, S. H. (1994). Routine ultrasonography *in utero* and speech development. *Ultrasound Obstet. Gynecol.,* **4**, 101–3

39. Kinnier-Wilson, I. M. and Waterhouse, J. A. H. (1984). Obstetric ultrasound and childhood malignancies. *Lancet,* **2**, 997–8

40. Cartwright, R. A., McKinney, P. A., Hopton, P. A., Birch, J. M., Hartley, A. L., Mann, J. R., Waterhouse, J. A. H., Johnston, H. E., Draper, G. J. and Stiller, C. (1984). Ultrasound examinations in pregnancy and childhood cancer. *Lancet,* **2**, 999–1000

41. Hartley, A. L., Birch, J. M., McKinney, P. A., Teare, M. D., Blair, V., Carrette, J., Mann, J. R., Draper, G. J., Stiller, C. A., Johnston, H. S., Cartwright, R. A. and Waterhouse, J. A. H. (1988). The Inter-Regional Epidemiological Study of Childhood Cancer (IRESCC): case control study of children with bone and soft tissue sarcoma. *Br. J. Cancer,* **58**, 838–42

42. Buckely, J. D., Sather, H., Ruccione, K., Rogers, P. C., Haas, J. E., Henderson, B. E. and Hammond, G. D. (1989). A case control study of risk factors for hepatoblastoma: a report from the Children's Cancer Study Group. *Cancer,* **64**, 1169–76

43. Shu, X. O., Jin, F., Linet, M. S., Zheng, W., Clemens, J., Mills, J. and Gao, Y. T. (1994). Diagnostic X-ray and ultrasound exposure and risk of childhood cancer. *Br. J. Cancer,* **70**, 531–6

44. Luck, C. A. (1992). Value of routine ultrasound scanning at 19 weeks: a four year study of 8,849 deliveries. *Br. Med. J.,* **304**, 1474–8

Cost-effectiveness of routine ultrasound in pregnancy

11

D. A. Ellwood

SUMMARY

Routine ultrasound examination in the first half of pregnancy improves the detection rate of multiple pregnancies and reduces the rate of induction of labor for post-term pregnancy. The only measurable benefit to perinatal outcome is the detection of major fetal malformations which leads to pregnancy termination and a subsequent reduction in perinatal mortality. It would appear, therefore, that the principal benefits stem from accurate pregnancy dating. There is little indication that routine ultrasound in the second half of pregnancy leads to any measurable improvement in outcome. Although detection of the small-for-gestational age (SGA) fetus is enhanced, outcome is not improved. Indeed, this may lead to more frequent interventions such as induction of labor. There are no data to support the routine use of umbilical artery Doppler. The potential benefits of placentography require further study.

It can be concluded that, despite many attempts at using randomized, controlled trials of ultrasound at various stages, the evidence that routine ultrasound improves pregnancy outcome remains elusive. The major benefits in terms of pregnancy management stem from early diagnosis of twins and better gestational age determination, both of which may lead to more cost-effective approaches to obstetric intervention. Any cost saving attributable to fetal abnormality detection will be the result of termination of pregnancy, or decisions not to intervene in the neonatal period. Further information on current detection rates of major abnormalities is needed to enable an accurate assessment to be made of this benefit.

INTRODUCTION

In most developed countries it has become an accepted part of antenatal care that women will have at least one ultrasound examination during the course of their pregnancy. The most frequent use of routine obstetric ultrasound is the second-trimester morphology scan, usually performed at 18–20 weeks' gestation[1]. However, there are other occasions when ultrasound is used routinely, such as in the first trimester for dating or establishing fetal viability, or the third trimester for the assessment of fetal growth. Due to the high cost of ultrasound equipment, and the need for highly trained and skilled sonographers, ultrasound examination in pregnancy is relatively expensive. If all of the 250 000 women who give birth in Australia each year had a single examination, the cost estimate is approximately $25 million, assuming each examination has a real economic cost of $100. The available Australian data[2] suggest that many women have more than one ultrasound examination, and the average per pregnancy is approximately 1.3. Whilst some of the additional examinations may be for specific indications, many will be essentially routine screening in either the first or second trimester. In the UK, a recent survey indicated that more than one-third of hospital ultrasound units routinely offer women at least two scans in pregnancy[3].

Owing to the high cost of this intervention in relation to other components of antenatal care, it is essential to examine critically the cost-effectiveness of routine obstetric ultrasound. Whilst the cost of the examination can be estimated with reasonable certainty, the measurement of benefit in terms of pregnancy outcome is much more difficult. Nevertheless, there is a large number of studies in the literature which have attempted to evaluate the effect on perinatal outcome of various forms of obstetric ultrasound. By examining the proven benefits, it should be possible to perform a cost–benefit analysis.

ROUTINE ULTRASOUND APPLICATIONS

First-trimester ultrasound

Although first-trimester ultrasound examination is not recommended as part of routine antenatal care, it is widely performed and therefore must be included in any comprehensive review. Whilst it is often for specific indications such as uncertain dates, bleeding in early pregnancy, or poor correlation between uterine size and gestational age, the frequency with which it is used constitutes a *de facto* screening approach. There are no randomized, controlled trials in the literature of first-trimester screening ultrasound, but a recent publication has attempted to examine the possible benefits of a routine approach[4]. In this study it was shown that nearly 50% of women who underwent an examination at their first antenatal visit could have derived some potential benefit from the examination. These were the correction of gestational age, diagnosis of multiple or non-viable pregnancy and referral to a high-risk clinic because of uterine abnormality. These potential benefits for women need to be evaluated further by a randomized, controlled trial of first-trimester ultrasound examination in the antenatal clinic.

Second-trimester ultrasound

The primary purpose of a routine second-trimester examination has changed over the last 10–15 years, in line with the significant improvements in ultrasound equipment and sonography skills. Whilst the original purpose of this examination was to confirm gestational age or identify multiple pregnancies, the focus has shifted towards the detection of fetal abnormalities. The timing of the routine second-trimester examination at 18–20 weeks is essentially a compromise between the time that gives reasonable accuracy for gestational age assessment, and the ideal time for examining fetal structural development. The published data on randomized controlled trials span a period from 1982 to 1994. Because of the change in emphasis of diagnostic ultrasound, meaningful comparison is difficult.

In 1982, results were published of a randomized controlled trial of over 1000 pregnant women who all had a fetal biparietal diameter measurement performed at approximately 16 weeks' menstrual age[5]. The primary outcomes were perinatal mortality, birth weight for gestational age and Apgar score at 1 min. There were no significant differences in perinatal outcome based on these criteria, suggesting that routine dating at this stage did not improve pregnancy outcome. This was despite the fact that nearly 20% of women in this study had their dates corrected on the basis of their ultrasound examination. In 1984 a study in Norway considered a two-stage screening process in which women were randomly selected for ultrasound at 19 and 32 weeks of pregnancy[6]. Earlier diagnosis of twin pregnancy and fewer inductions for post-dates was reported in the screened group. One possible adverse outcome was that women who were screened were admitted to hospital more often, and would thus have incurred additional costs. These authors concluded that there were only marginal benefits in terms of pregnancy outcome from ultrasound screening, but advocated larger prospective studies. Another Scandinavian study of nearly 5000 women involved a trial of one-stage ultrasound screening at 15 weeks' gestation[7] and showed a reduction in the rate of induced labor, particularly for post-term pregnancies. Earlier detection of twins was noted, but no measurable effect on perinatal outcome occurred. A slightly increased mean birth weight in the women who were screened was suggested to result from reduced smoking in pregnancy encouraged in those women at ultrasound examination. Ewigman and co-workers[8] reported on a randomized controlled trial of ultrasound at 12–18 weeks in over 900 women examined for assessment of gestational age, rather than detection of fetal abnormality. This study also showed no measurable benefit, despite altering the estimated date of confinement for a quarter of the patients offered routine ultrasound.

The Helsinki Ultrasound trial[9], reported in 1990, was the first randomized trial that specifically addressed the question of fetal abnormality detection. In this study over 9000 women were randomized to receive ultrasound screening at 16–18 weeks at two sites. This study showed a significant reduction in perinatal mortality in the groups that were screened. The nearly 50% reduction was mainly due to improved detection of lethal fetal malformations, leading to induced abortion.

From the studies discussed so far it would appear that routine ultrasound examination in the first half of pregnancy can lead to better assessment of gestational age, earlier detection of multiple pregnancies and improved detection of fetal malformations at a time when it is possible to proceed to termination of pregnancy. A recent meta-analysis of these five trials[10] clearly demonstrated the improved detection of twins before 26 weeks and a reduction in the rate of induction of labor for post-term pregnancy (Table 1). There was also an apparent reduction in admission to special care nurseries and in the rate of low birth weight infants (< 2500 g), although only in singleton pregnancies. It is interesting to note that there were no measurable effects in twin pregnancies despite the earlier diagnosis. Although the Helsinki trial showed an improvement in perinatal mortality, this effect was not present when all trials were included in the meta-analysis, and this presumably reflects the relatively poor performance in the earlier trials of ultrasound for fetal malformation detection. During the 13-year period of these trials there have been significant improvements in ultrasound technology and sonography. The most obvious benefits of routine ultrasound examination in early pregnancy come from more accurate gestational age dating and it should be noted that this can be achieved at an earlier stage in pregnancy than the current timing of 18–20 weeks. The justification for later screening, and the additional costs involved for a more comprehensive examination, must come from improved detection of fetal malformations.

There are a number of non-randomized prospective studies in the literature which may give some indication of the expected sensitivity for the detection of fetal abnormalities in using good equipment, following establishment protocols and using trained sonographers and sonologists. In 1992, a 4-year study was reported from the UK in which an ultrasound department offered screening to nearly 9000 women, with a 96% acceptance rate. The sensitivity for fetal anomalies at 19 weeks was 85%, although this figure is based on all anomalies and includes a large proportion of relatively minor structural defects[11]. Another report from the UK showed a similar high detection rate from one center[12]. Perhaps a more realistic appraisal of abnormality detection in an unselected population comes from examining two collaborative studies reported in 1991 and 1993. The Belgian Multi-centric study[13] requested data from four sites, collected between 1984 and 1989. This study showed correct detection of only 40% of the 2.3% of structurally abnormal fetuses, and only 21% were diagnosed before 23 weeks' gestation. A similar study in northern England[14] reported a figure of 50%. Although detection rates (sensitivity) in these two studies were low, the

Table 1 The effects of routine ultrasound examination in early pregnancy (five trials reviewed). Data from reference 9. Only outcomes that reached statistical significance have been included

	Number of trials	Odds ratio	95% CI
Termination of pregnancy for fetal abnormalities	1	7.29	2.23–23.79
Twins undiagnosed at 26 weeks	4	0.15	0.04–0.50
Induction for post-term pregnancy	3	0.60	0.46–0.79
Admission to special care	3	0.83	0.70–0.98
Low birth weight (< 2500 g) in singletons	3	0.61	0.47–0.79

specificity in both was higher than 99%. A recent publication specifically addressed this question and gave a relatively reassuring view of the accuracy of the diagnosis[15].

One problem of interpretation of these data is that these studies included patients screened over a period from 1984 to 1992, and since then there have been many significant improvements in the ability to detect major structural malformations with ultrasound. It has to be acknowledged that the accuracy of ultrasound in 1997 is not known, using state-of-the art equipment, trained sonographers and modern protocols. It is also important to realize that 'best practice' results in this field do not reflect the expected average detection rates from all sites using a variety of equipment and sonographer skill levels (the 'real world'). These facts emphasize the need for continued appraisal of the performance of routine second-trimester ultrasound in the detection of fetal abnormalities.

Third-trimester ultrasound

In standard clinical practice, third-trimester ultrasound examinations are usually performed for a specific indication. However, there have been a number of trials addressing the question of routine ultrasound examination to improve perinatal outcome in low-risk pregnancies. These trials have looked at three specific areas: diagnosis of SGA fetuses, Doppler ultrasound for the detection of increased placental vascular resistance and routine placentography.

Screening for SGA fetuses

Two trials reported in 1984 employed two-stage screening and used as an endpoint the diagnosis of the SGA fetus. The first trial in just under 900

women showed improved detection of SGA fetuses, but no improvement in outcome, although the authors acknowledged that the numbers were probably too small to show any significant benefit in a low-risk population[16]. In the same year a Norwegian study showed that two-stage screening led to more frequent diagnosis of SGA fetuses, and these mothers received more active treatment in terms of admission and number of days spent in hospital[6]. However, there were no measurable improvements in perinatal outcome. A later study from Denmark showed that revealing ultrasound results in apparently SGA fetuses did not improve outcome in terms of morbidity, but led to more frequent induction of labour[17]. The most recent study, also from Denmark, included 1000 pregnant women who had early pregnancy dating with ultrasound, and a follow-up scan at 28 weeks and every 3rd week after that[18]. This approach significantly increased the diagnosis of SGA fetuses, and of elective deliveries, but there were no measurable improvements in neonatal morbidity or mortality.

When a meta-analysis was performed of these trials, there were no demonstrable differences between the groups who had ultrasound screening and those who either were not screened, or did not have their results revealed (Table 2)[19]. The conclusion from the analysis of these trials is that there is no support for routine ultrasound biometry in late pregnancy[6].

Routine Doppler ultrasound screening

Doppler ultrasound examination of umbilical artery blood flow is now widely used in the monitoring and management of high-risk pregnancies. In theory, the ability of this investigation to predict fetal growth retardation could be used

Table 2 Routine fetal athropometry in late pregnancy (four trials reviewed). Data from reference 19

	Number of trials	Odds ratio	95% CI
Antenatal admission	3	1.32	1.10–1.59
Labor induction	4	1.20	0.98–1.47
Low Apgar score	4	1.06	0.79–1.42
Special care admission	3	1.29	0.95–1.75
Perinatal death	4	0.98	0.34–2.81

to identify the at-risk fetus in a low-risk population. There are two published randomized, controlled trials that have evaluated routine Doppler ultrasound in the third trimester. The only significant result in a study of approximately 2500 women was an increased rate of perinatal death in the group that received monthly Doppler ultrasound examinations (both umbilical and uterine arteries)[20]. Another similar sized study showed no changes in obstetric intervention rates or short-term neonatal morbidity following Doppler ultrasound screening at 28 and 34 weeks[21]. A meta-analysis of the results of these two trials and one unreported study shows no improvement in pregnancy outcome with routine Doppler ultrasound screening[22].

It is clear from published data in high-risk women that Doppler ultrasound performs well in prediction of fetal hypoxia and acidosis. The inability of Doppler to improve outcome in low-risk women would suggest that there is little prospect for any test of fetal well-being or placental function to have a significant impact on pregnancy outcome in this group.

Routine placentography

Placentography is the use of ultrasound imaging of placental appearances to predict adverse pregnancy outcome[23]. Placental 'grading' using a defined measure of placental maturity based on appearance was used in a randomized trial of ultrasound at 30–32 and 34–36 weeks[24]. Revealing results of placental grading apparently improved pregnancy outcome using a number of measures of perinatal morbidity, including meconium staining of the liquor, Apgar score at 5 min and perinatal death. This study is the only one in the literature which shows strong evidence of improved perinatal outcome based on a third-trimester ultrasound technique. This approach needs to be further examined in larger studies.

RECENT STUDIES

Two large randomized controlled trials have been reported in the last 2 years which have examined the effect of ultrasound on perinatal outcome. The first of these is the Routine Antenatal Diagnostic Imaging with Ultrasound (RADIUS) trial[25] which was reported in late 1993. The second is a study from Western Australia in which women were randomized to receive frequent ultrasound and continuous wave Doppler studies of the umbilical artery on five occasions between 18 weeks and term[26]. Owing to the magnitude and importance of these two studies they will be discussed in detail.

The RADIUS trial

This was a multicenter trial involving over 15 000 pregnant women who were considered to be at low risk for abnormal perinatal outcome[25]. Following randomization they were assigned to either the ultrasound screening group, or a control group. The screened group had examinations performed at 15–22 weeks, and again at 31–35 weeks. Those in the control group only had examinations for specific medical indications. All studies were performed in one of 28 ultrasound laboratories participating in the RADIUS trial and some attempt was made at standardization of equipment and protocols used.

The mean number of examinations was higher for women in the screened group (2.2) than those in the control group (0.6). Adverse perinatal outcome was defined as perinatal death, or neonatal morbidity, which covered a wide range of adverse outcomes. There was no difference in adverse outcomes, rates of preterm delivery and distribution of birth weights between the two groups. There was a significant difference in the detection of major fetal anomalies between the two groups, but the sensitivity for ultrasound detection was low, being 35% in total and only 17% before 24 weeks. The authors of the RADIUS trial concluded that ultrasound screening in low-risk women does not improve perinatal outcome, and that the use of routine ultrasound screening in the USA would add considerably to the cost of care in pregnancy.

The RADIUS trial has been criticized for many reasons. It has been claimed that the use of specific eligibility and exclusion criteria has resulted in a study population that was at such low risk for adverse perinatal outcome that the trial could not have been expected to show any significant improvement. A further criticism is that the number of sites used may have resulted in many scans being performed by relatively inexperienced sonographers or sonologists. The overall low rate of detection of fetal anomalies is perhaps an indication that the quality of the ultrasound screening was suboptimal. When compared with previous trials, it is noteworthy that many patients in whom ultrasound dating could have been beneficial were specifically excluded, such as those with an irregular menstrual cycle, or conception whilst taking the oral contraceptive pill. Many of the apparent benefits from the earlier trials would relate to establishment or confirmation of gestational age.

Frequent ultrasound examination during pregnancy

This study of nearly 3000 women in Western Australia questioned the benefit of multiple examinations with ultrasound (both biometry and Doppler) at 18, 24, 28, 34 and 38 weeks gestation[26]. An intensively screened randomized population was compared with a group that was exposed to B-mode imaging only at 18 weeks of pregnancy. This study showed no improvement in perinatal outcome, but apparently showed an increase in the rate of SGA fetuses in the intensively exposed group, raising the possibility that frequent exposure to ultrasound may have influenced fetal growth. The results of this trial have been reported in detail elsewhere in this book (see Chapter 10). In terms of this attempt at cost–benefit analysis, it is important to emphasize that the use of frequent ultrasound did not improve perinatal outcome. Because of the possible effect on fetal growth, the authors concluded that it would be prudent to limit ultrasound examinations of the fetus to those cases in which the information is likely to be of clinical importance.

COST–BENEFIT ANALYSIS

In summarizing the results of the trials reported to date, a number of statements can be made. Routine ultrasound examination in the first half of pregnancy clearly improves the detection rate of multiple pregnancies, and also reduces the rate of induction of labor for post-term pregnancy, presumably by more accurate dating. The only measurable beneficial effect on perinatal outcome appears to be the detection of major fetal malformations which then leads to pregnancy termination and a subsequent reduction in perinatal mortality. It would appear, therefore, that the major benefits may stem from the ascertainment of accurate pregnancy dating. Whether this should be performed in the first trimester, at which stage ultrasound dating can be very quick, or in the second trimester as part of a fetal anomaly scan is an important part of any cost–benefit analysis. The additional time, and more sophisticated equipment and protocols used for the second-trimester scan, can be justified in an economic sense only if the increased benefit attributable to fetal anomaly detection leads to a significant reduction in costs. Some of these costs may relate to the ongoing care of a handicapped child, but the available data would suggest that ultrasound performs best in relation to the detection of lethal malformations.

There is little indication that routine ultrasound examination in the second half of pregnancy leads to any measurable improvement in outcome. Although there is an improvement in the ability to detect the SGA fetus, this does not improve outcome. Indeed, this may lead to more frequent intervention such as induction of labor. There are no available data to support the routine use of umbilical artery Doppler, but placentography should be further studied.

Whilst the cost side of the equation can be determined fairly accurately, and costs per patient of routine screening factored into the costs of antenatal care, the apparent benefits from the studies reported to date are more difficult to quantify. The cost reductions could come from reducing hospital admission, reducing intervention such as induction of labor and operative delivery, and reducing time spent in neonatal nurseries due to iatrogenic prematurity. The only way to obtain accurate information in a way that has local relevance is to conduct a trial of ultrasound use in which the costs of intervention, which are related to ultrasound diagnosis or to the absence of information which would have been provided by ultrasound, can be collected prospectively. One other potential benefit of routine ultrasound examination in pregnancy stems from the argument that the ability of ultrasound to perform well in high-risk patients is enhanced by the use of ultrasound in the low-risk setting. The ability to recognize deviations from normal may be significantly better in units that are used to a high volume throughput of routine examinations.

CONCLUSIONS

Despite many attempts using randomized, controlled trials of ultrasound scanning at various stages, the evidence that routine ultrasound examination improves pregnancy outcome remains elusive. The major benefits in terms of pregnancy management stem from early diagnosis of twins and more accurate gestational age determination, both of which may lead to more cost-effective approaches to obstetric intervention. Any cost saving attributable to fetal abnormality detection will be the result of termination of pregnancy, or decisions not to intervene in the neonatal period. Further information on current detection rates of major abnormalities is needed to enable an accurate assessment to be made of this benefit.

References

1. O'Brien, G. D., Robinson, H. P. and Warren, P. (1993). The 18 to 20 weeks obstetrical scan. *Med. J. Aust.*, **158**, 567–70
2. Yates, J. M., Lumley, J. and Bell, R. J. (1995). The prevalence and timing of obstetric ultrasound in Victoria 1991–1992; a population based study. *Aust. N. Z. J. Obstet. Gynaecol.*, **35**, 375–9
3. Hay, S. and McLean, E. (1994). *The Timing and Content of Routine Obstetric Ultrasound in the UK.* (London: College of Radiographers)
4. Peek, M. J., Devonald, K. J., Beilby, R. and Ellwood, D. A. (1994). The value of routine early pregnancy ultrasound in the antenatal booking clinic. *Aust. NZ Obstet. Gynaecol.*, **34**, 140–3
5. Bennet, M. J., Little, G., Dewhurst, J. and Chamberlain, G. (1982). Predictive value of ultrasound in early pregnancy: a randomised controlled trial. *Br. J. Obstet. Gynaecol.*, **89**, 338–41
6. Bakketeig, L. S., Eik-Nes, S. H., Jacobsen, G., Ulstein, M. K., Brodtkorb, C. J., Balstad, P., Eriksen, B. C. and Jorgensen, N. P. (1984). Randomised controlled trial of ultrasonographic screening in pregnancy. *Lancet*, **2**, 207–11
7. Waldenstrom, U., Axelsson, O., Nilsson, S., Ekwind, G., Ole, F. and Lindeberg, S. (1988). Effects of routine one-stage ultrasound screening in pregnancy; a randomised controlled trial. *Lancet*, **2**, 585–8
8. Ewigman, B., Lefevre, M. and Hesser, J. (1990). A randomised trial of routine prenatal ultrasound. *Obstet. Gynecol.*, **76**, 189–94
9. Saari-Kemppainen, A., Karjalainen, O., Yiöstalo, P. and Heinonen, O. P. (1990). Ultrasound screening and perinatal mortality: controlled trial of systematic one-stage screening in pregnancy. *Lancet*, **336**, 387–91
10. Neilson, J. P. (1994). Routine ultrasound in early pregnancy. In Enkin, M. W., Keirse, M. J. N. C., Renfrew, M. J. and Neilson, J. P. (eds.) *Pregnancy and Childbirth Module. Cochrane Database of Systematic Reviews*, Review No. 03872, Cochrane updates on disk. (Oxford: Update Software)
11. Luck, C. A. (1992). Value of routine ultrasound screening at 19 weeks: a four year study of 8,849 deliveries. *Br. Med. J.,* **304**, 1474–8
12. Chitty, L. S., Hunt, G. H., Moore, J. and Lobb, M. O. (1991). Effectiveness of routine ultrasonography in detecting fetal structural abnormalities in a low risk population. *Br. Med. J.*, **303**, 1165–9
13. Levi, S., Hyjaz, Y., Schaaps, J. P., Defoort, P., Coulon, R. and Buckens, P. (1991). Sensitivity and specificity of routine antenatal screening for congenital anomalies by ultrasound: the Belgian Multicentric Study. *Ultrasound Obstet. Gynecol.*, **1**, 102–10

14. Bucher, H. C. and Schmidt, J. C. (1993). Does routine ultrasound improve outcome in pregnancy? Meta-analysis of various outcomes. *Br. Med. J.,* **307**, 13–17

15. Brend, I. R., Kaminopetros, P., Cave, M., Irving, M. C. and Lilford, R. J. (1994). Specificity of antenatal ultrasound in the Yorkshire Region: a propective study of 2261 ultrasound detected anomalies. *Br. J. Obstet. Gynaecol.,* **101**, 392–7

16. Neilson, J. P., Munjanja, S. P. and Whitfield, C. R. (1984). Screening for small for dates fetuses: a controlled trial. *Br. Med. J.,* **289**, 1179–82

17. Secher, N. J., Hansen, P. K., Enstrup, C., Sindberg Eriksen, P. and Morsing, G. (1987). A randomised study of fetal abdominal diameter and fetal weight estimation for detection of light-for-gestational infants in low-risk pregnancies. *Br. J. Obstet. Gynaecol.,* **94**, 105–9

18. Larsen, T., Larsen, J. K., Petersen, S. and Greisen, G. (1992). Detection of small-for-gestational age fetuses by ultrasound screening in a high risk population: a randomised controlled study. *Br. J. Obstet. Gynaecol.,* **99**, 469–74

19. Neilson, J. P. (1994). Routine fetal anthropometry in late pregnancy. In Enkin, M. W., Keirse, M. J. N. C., Renfrew, M. J. and Neilson, J. P. (eds.) *Pregnancy and Childbirth Module. Cochrane Database of Systematic Reviews,* Review No. 03873, Cochrane updates on disk. (Oxford: Update Software)

20. Davies, J. A., Gallivan, S. and Spencer, J. A. D. (1992). Randomised controlled trial of Doppler ultrasound screening of placental perfusion during pregnancy. *Lancet,* **340**, 1299–303

21. Mason, G. C., Lilford, R. J., Porter, J., Nelson, E. and Tyrell, S. (1993). Randomised comparison of routine versus highly selective use of Doppler ultrasound in low risk pregnancies. *Br. J. Obstet. Gynaecol.,* **100**, 130–3

22. Neilson, J. P. (1994). Routine Doppler ultrasound screening of unselected pregnancies. In Enkin, M. W., Keirse, M. J. N. C., Renfrew, M. J. and Neilson, J. P. (eds.) *Pregnancy and Childbirth Module. Cochrane Database of Systematic Reviews,* Review No. 07357, Cochrane updates on disk. (Oxford: Update Software)

23. Grannum, P. A., Berkowitz, R. L. and Hobbins, J. C. (1979). The ultrasonic changes in the maturing placenta and their relation to fetal pulmonary maturity. *Am. J. Obstet. Gynaecol.,* **133**, 915–22

24. Proud, J. and Grant, A. M. (1987). Third trimester placental grading by ultrasonography as a test of fetal well-being. *Br. Med. J.,* **294**, 1641–7

25. Ewigman, B. G., Crane, J. P., Frigoletto, F. D., LeFevre, M. L., Bain, R. P., McNellies, D. and the RADIUS Study Group (1993). Effect of prenatal ultrasound screening on perinatal outcome. *N. Engl. J. Med.,* **329**, 821–7

26. Newnham, J. P., Evans, S. F., Michael, C. A., Stanley, F. J. and Landau, L. I. (1993). Effect of frequent ultrasound during pregnancy: a randomised controlled trial. *Lancet,* **342**, 887–91

Regulations, recommendations and safety guidelines

12

S. B. Barnett and G. Kossoff

SUMMARY

The regulatory process that controls acoustic output from ultrasound medical devices has been largely dictated by the Food and Drug Administration (FDA) in the USA, empowered by an act of Congress. In recent years there have been significant changes that make the development of an internationally acceptable standard on ultrasound safety both complicated and imperative. The trend towards self-regulation has resulted in a move away from the relatively simple, but outdated, scheme of enforced application-specific limits on acoustic output. The FDA now provides an option for manufacturers to obtain market approval for medical ultrasound devices that can increase the intensity at the fetus by almost a factor of 8, provided that an output display is incorporated into the equipment design. Meanwhile, the International Electrotechnical Commission is developing international standards for the measurement of acoustic output and for the classification of medical equipment, by its acoustic fields, into categories that either are without risk or require a form of display of risk of producing a recognized biophysical effect.

The combination of recent changes in the regulation of medical ultrasound and continuing developments in international standards will allow greater control by the ultrasonologist of higher output power levels used in diagnostic equipment. Major national ultrasound societies have formulated guidelines for the safe use of ultrasound in medicine. There is a strong need for continuing education to ensure that appropriate risk/benefit assessments are made by ultrasonologists based on an understanding of the probability of biological effects occurring with each type of ultrasound procedure. The relaxation of intensity limits for pre-market approval by the FDA allows substantially increased intensity of ultrasound to be delivered to the fetus. Modern diagnostic equipment operating at maximum output conditions can produce significant biological effects in mammalian tissues. These issues have been addressed by the World Federation for Ultrasound in Medicine and Biology in published conclusions and recommendations that represent international consensus on safe use of ultrasound in medicine.

INTRODUCTION

To regulate or educate? That is an interesting question that relates to the safe use of ultrasound in medicine. Is it better to limit the acoustic output by law or to rely on optimum patient exposure based on informed use?

Most national ultrasound societies have a safety committee whose role is to provide information on the risk of bioeffects and to issue safety guidelines. Examples of policy statements are given later in this chapter. Information on bioeffects and safety is also disseminated through presentations at various ultrasound conferences. However, the relatively low levels of audience attendance at some of these presentations suggests that the concept of voluntary attention to safety issues may not be appropriate or effective. The situation is made more difficult by the unknown quantity of ultrasonologists who practice outside tertiary centers and who do not have any affiliation with ultrasound societies. As authors of this current volume on safety of ultrasound in obstetrics and gynecology, it is our sincere hope that the majority of users of ultrasound equipment will have access to the latest information presented in this book.

Medical ultrasonography continues to enjoy increasingly widespread use as an effective diagnostic clinical tool. Improvements in resolution and image quality and in gray-scale definition have been particularly important in obstetrics. The results have been further enhanced with the advent of endovaginal examinations which allow direct access to anatomical structures and visualization of the embryo or fetus without suffering the beam-interference effects, or ultrasound attenuation, caused by overlying abdominal skin, fat and musculature. Pulsed Doppler spectral flow analysis and color Doppler imaging techniques offer the potential to increase diagnostic effectiveness and may be attractive for applications in early pregnancy.

Developments in recent years may have a significant impact on the way in which ultrasound is used. The emphasis is changing from one of regulation to that of allowing the clinician or ultrasound technologist control of substantially higher acoustic exposures based on the assessment of the risk/benefit ratio for each type of examination. It is appropriate that clinicians take the responsibility of risk assessment based on information on bioeffects provided by the scientific community and equipment output conditions provided by the manufacturer. Clearly, the risk/benefit ratio changes significantly according to the medical reason for undertaking each type of ultrasonographic examination. Routine scans may have low benefit and could present a risk in certain fetal examinations, depending on the exposure conditions chosen and the sensitivity of the tissues being insonated. In addition, both the benefit and the risk depend largely on the skill and competence of the ultrasonologist. It is essential that users of ultrasound equipment have an understanding of bioeffects mechanisms and are cognizant of the potential risks in different modes of operation.

HISTORICAL PERSPECTIVE

The imaging and measurement capabilities of diagnostic ultrasound devices have evolved over the past 30 years to allow discrimination of fine detail and improved diagnostic sensitivity in modern equipment. It has also been shown (see Chapter 3) that the development of sophisticated ultrasound equipment has been accompanied by substantial increases in acoustic output. In recent years there has been an increasing trend in some countries to use ultrasound at early stages of embryonic development.

A current topic of debate is whether or not there is risk, or benefit, associated with routine use of pulsed Doppler ultrasound during the first trimester in uncomplicated pregnancy. For original B-mode imaging equipment this was not an issue for consideration, because (1) the bistable (black and white only) images relied on the different acoustic impedance between soft tissue and bone that occurs in the second and third trimesters; and (2) the acoustic output was low compared with that available today. Improvements in technology have allowed both increased output power of transducers and measurement sensitivity of measuring hydrophones, thereby showing the higher acoustic intensities emitted by current diagnostic devices.

In the early 1970s major national ultrasound societies were established to explore applications of ultrasound in clinical medicine. It was also acknowledged that there was a need to study the safety aspects of ultrasound exposures. In those early days of ultrasonography, scientific research into biological effects used imaging devices with modest acoustic outputs and researchers had difficulty in finding biological endpoints that were sufficiently sensitive to respond. The Bioeffects Committee of the American Institute of Ultrasound in Medicine (AIUM) was the first to publish authoritative statements on bioeffects and safety. In 1976 the AIUM published the conclusions of a review of the early scientific literature. The specific wording has been carefully modified in succeeding years, but its essence is that there was no evidence of independently confirmed significant adverse biological effects in mammalian tissue exposed *in vivo* to intensities below 100 mW/cm^2 (spatial peak temporal average intensity, I_{SPTA})[1]. The situation has changed in the 1990s with the reports of lung capillary bleeding in animals following exposure to diagnostic levels of ultrasound[2].

In 1976, another significant event involved the inaugural meeting of the World Federation for Ultrasound in Medicine and Biology (WFUMB), in San Francisco. The WFUMB has since evolved into a large international organization. During the past 11 years the WFUMB has demonstrated a serious commitment to establishing conclusions and recommendations on safety based on international scientific consensus. It has done this by sponsoring a number of symposia on standardization and safety of ultrasound in medicine. This is described in more detail later in this chapter.

Only in recent years, i.e. in the 1990s, has it been seriously considered that diagnostic applications of ultrasound might produce significant biological effects. Major ultrasound societies and organizations have paid attention to the safety of diagnostic ultrasound and progress has been achieved towards identifying international consensus on important issues. In recent years, knowledge on biophysical effects of ultrasound has become a fundamental consideration in the process of setting international standards for safety of ultrasound in medicine, an important function of the International Electrotechnical Commission (IEC).

In the past there has been little regulation of the clinical use of ultrasound, with a corresponding lack of international safety standards or requirements for calibrating output from diagnostic equipment. The only effective regulatory body is the FDA (Food and Drug Administration, Center for Devices and Radiological Health, USA) which introduced, somewhat arbitrarily, limits on acoustic output for equipment sold within the USA. The approved intensity limits were based on pre-enactment maximum levels of equipment manufactured in 1976 and from which no adverse effects had been reported. A Medical Devices Amendment to the Food and Drug Act, enacted by the US Congress in May 1976, provided the process for approving medical devices for marketing on the basis of the manufacturers' ability to demonstrate substantial equivalence (in safety and efficacy of each new device) to devices on the market prior to the enactment date. The FDA enforced application-specific limits on equipment output[3]. The permissible limit was lowest for ophthalmic (17 mW/cm^2 I_{SPTA}) and fetal (94 mW/cm^2 I_{SPTA}) exposures, where the tissue target is more sensitive to damage.

There are some difficulties associated with the original FDA approach, known as the 510(k) process of compliance. The limits on acceptable levels for equipment output were based on assumptions about the safety of existing (pre-1976) equipment rather than an understanding of the mechanisms by which biological effects are produced. Medical ultrasound technology and its applications have changed since 1976, together with substantial changes in acoustic characteristics of the delivered pulsed ultrasound. Research has produced significant developments in the understanding of specific mechanisms of biological effects. The advent of duplex pulsed Doppler ultrasound systems has led to substantial increases in power outputs of diagnostic equipment[4], as described in Chapter 3. The maximum output levels available in certain modes of operation (pulsed Doppler examinations of deep vessels or subcostal cardiography in adults) are capable of depositing significant amounts of heat in biological tissues.

In 1993 the AIUM in conjunction with the National Electrical Manufacturers Association (NEMA) developed a voluntary scheme for on-screen labelling of diagnostic ultrasound devices, known as the Output Display Standard[5].

After almost 20 years the FDA has, in essence, altered its emphasis on application-specific intensity limits for pre-market approval of equipment in the USA. There is now an option whereby substantially increased I_{SPTA} intensity levels may be delivered to the fetus, or the eye, provided that the equipment incorporates a visual indicator of its output and likelihood of risk of producing biological effects. By using equipment with an output display, far greater responsibility is placed on the users of these devices to determine patient exposure levels and potentially greater diagnostic capability. Because of uncertainties in measured acoustic output and the estimated *in situ* dosimetry, these output display indices are intended as a guide to the risk of inducing certain biological effects rather than providing absolute values of acoustic output or related biophysical parameters.

EQUIPMENT OUTPUT DISPLAYS

The FDA Center for Devices and Radiological Health agreed to incorporate the AIUM/NEMA Output Display Standard (ODS) as a part of the FDA's pre-market approval process. These indicators are expressed in terms which reflect the potential for thermal and non-thermal biological effects. Whilst agreeing to adopt the AIUM/NEMA Output Display Standard as an option to replace the system of application-specific limits, the FDA has maintained an overall maximum output limit of 720 mW/cm^2 for all equipment[6]. Table 1 illustrates the increased available ultrasound exposure in terms of spatial peak temporal average intensity for equipment using the conventional application-specific FDA limits compared with the track 3 Output Display option for current, high-output devices.

High-output devices can be approved by the FDA for use in the USA with a maximum I_{SPTA} output of 720 mW/cm^2 for all applications, as long as a thermal index (TI) and mechanical index (MI) are displayed for every possible setting of transducer type, output setting, focus, frame rate and pulse rate. Consequently, for fetal applications the allowable maximum

derated I_{SPTA} intensity can be increased by a factor of 8 if the ultrasonographer chooses to use the highest available output. A potential 42-fold increase in the maximum allowed I_{SPTA} could be applied in ophthalmic applications, but the MI must be kept below 0.23. The implications for clinical practice are that all users must be aware of the exposure capabilities of these new, high-output devices. There are no automatic safeguards for the output of machines that have an ODS set. The user can ensure safety only by keeping the thermal and mechanical indices as low as possible during all examinations. The development of these indices is described in detail elsewhere[7].

The Output Display Standard comprises a thermal and a mechanical index that is intended to give a warning of the risk that an extended exposure may produce a significant thermal or non-thermal bioeffect in human tissue. Temperature rise and cavitation are, in turn, dependent on acoustic factors such as total energy output, the mode, the shape of the ultrasound beam, the position of the focus, the center frequency, the shape of the waveform, the frame rate and the amount of time during which the beam produces energy. The TI and MI are each designed to take these factors into account, notifying the user about the potential for ultrasound-induced bioeffects.

The TI is a quantity that is related to an estimated temperature rise, and is the ratio of total acoustic power to the acoustic power that would be required to raise tissue temperature by 1 °C, under defined assumptions. Assumptions are made about an average value for ultrasonic attenuation for soft tissue. The important acoustic parameters are beamwidth, average power and temporally and spatially averaged intensity. The TI gives a relative estimate of temperature rise at a specific point along the ultrasound beam. This index cannot be assumed to give the actual increase in temperature for all possible conditions, because the assumed conditions for heating in tissue are too complex. A TI of 2 represents a higher temperature rise than a TI of 1, but not necessarily a rise of 2 °C. Thus, a theoretical estimate is obtained, based on assumptions about the exposure conditions of

Table 1 Comparison of maximum allowable spatial peak temporal average intensity (I_{SPTA}) limits for FDA-regulated application-specific and Output Display Standard (ODS) options. (Intensity derated by a value which corresponds to attenuation by the tissue path)

	I_{SPTA} *limit* (mW/cm^2)	*ODS track 3 option* (mW/cm^2)
Peripheral vessel	720	720
Cardiac	430	720
Fetal, neonatal	94	720
Ophthalmic	17	720

tissue properties for any particular examination condition. There are three specific thermal indices: TIS, thermal index for soft tissue; TIB, thermal index for bone; TIC, thermal index for cranial bone. The TIS is used to provide information concerning temperature rise within homogeneous soft tissue, the TIB gives information on temperature rise in bone at or near the focus of the beam and the TIC gives the temperature increase of bone at or near the surface, such as during a cranial examination.

The MI gives a relative indication of the potential for mechanical effects, such as cavitation (the violent collapse of a bubble in tissue). Therefore, the MI is required to be displayed for B-mode imaging. The potential for mechanical effects increases as the peak pressure increases and decreases as the frequency increases for scanning modes. That is probably more significant than thermal effects. According to FDA regulations, the MI can range up to 1.9 for all uses except ophthalmic, for which a maximum MI limit of 0.23 applies. The higher the index value, the higher the probability of a biological effect. The value of learning to implement the ALARA (as low as reasonably achievable) principle allows the use of TI and MI values that are as small as possible, while keeping the quality of the scan as high as possible.

The index that is displayed depends on the choice of transducer, and the mode of examination. For example, for B-mode imaging, the MI will be displayed. For Doppler, M-mode or color flow imaging, the TI will be displayed. Since there are three subcategories of TI (i.e. TIS, TIB and TIC), only one of these is required to be displayed at a time, but the machine must allow the user to retrieve the other two if needed. Only ultrasound systems capable of exceeding an MI or TI of 1 are required to display these indices at values beginning at 0.4 and ranging up to the maximum. Further information is available from the AIUM[8].

INTERNATIONAL STANDARDS/GUIDELINES

There are some important issues that need to be understood when considering the AIUM/ NEMA output labelling scheme. The duration of exposure is not included in the index of risk, and this remains an important consideration, particularly for thermal effects. The dwell time is an important aspect of the ALARA principle that is not incorporated in these output display indices. The user should remember that, besides the TI and MI being kept as low as possible, the total exposure time in any one location should be kept as short as possible.

Following its most recent safety symposium, the World Federation for Ultrasound in Medicine and Biology (WFUMB) issued a recommendation that, '. . . safety guidelines should include an appropriate duration factor'. This aspect of safety issues has been recognized by the International Electrotechnical Commission (IEC) in its deliberations toward developing international safety standards.

Furthermore, the TI does not take account of patient temperature. This may be an important consideration for obstetrics. A recommendation of the WFUMB[9] states,

> 'Care should be taken to avoid unnecessary additional embryonic and fetal risk from ultrasound examinations of febrile patients.'

Whilst it is generally agreed that the display of biophysical indices can provide useful information to the user, there are certain limitations in the AIUM/NEMA Output Display Standard. The European Committee for Ultrasound Radiation Safety (ECURS) has published an informative tutorial paper on the thermal and mechanical indices[10], which draws attention to some problems. As an example, it suggests that the models for deriving 'reasonable worst-case' exposures for the indices may not be adequate to describe first-trimester scanning through a full bladder where the attenuating effect of overlying tissue is small.

In addition to this, the purpose of the MI is to predict the likelihood of cavitation-type bioeffects where the peak amplitude in pressure is a critical parameter. The intended use is for the display of MI to be included in B-mode imaging. However, comparison between modes of operation demonstrates no difference of any significance between the pulse amplitudes. Chapter 3 of this book states: 'In the values tabulated, the median values vary from 2.1 MPa for pulsed Doppler to 2.4 MPa for imaging within an overall range spanning 0.45–5.54 MPa. This is an important observation, since a view has been held that pulse amplitude is an important exposure parameter only for imaging, and not for other applications. This assertion is not supported by the evidence reported in any survey.'

The IEC has developed an international standard (IEC 1157) that requires the declaration of acoustic outputs by manufacturers[11]. The standard provides an exemption for devices with low output: those producing peak negative acoustic pressure less than 1.0 MPa and I_{SPTA} less than 100 mW/cm^2. When the IEC standard is adopted by individual countries it will effectively ensure that manufacturers will need to declare a range of acoustic output parameters to the user. Some form of on-screen display may be the preferred option.

A safety classification standard is currently under development. In the approach taken by the IEC, equipment that is classified as safe, or Class A, will require no further attention, whereas Class B equipment is determined to pose some risk of bioeffects under some conditions of use. The equipment is to be classified according to the worst-case exposure condition within its acoustic field. Equipment that carries a B classification will require an approved form of output display to advise the user of the extent of risk for different applications.

SAFETY GUIDELINES

It has become evident that the power outputs of certain new equipment are approaching the thresholds for biological effects, particularly when the equipment is used in pulsed Doppler or duplex modes. Therefore, the concept of safety classification has been introduced. The new trend towards self-regulation will require users to make decisions about appropriate examination exposures on the basis of displayed equipment output. These displays will provide an indicator of dosage for each examination in each mode of operation, or whenever the output controls are altered. Some physical classifi-

cation of equipment will remain, for example to identify the transducers, or modes of application, that are not intended for fetal use.

The rationale behind the classification approaches is for a display to provide a reasonable worst-case indicator of potential bioeffects, which may stimulate the user to apply the ALARA (as low as reasonably achievable) principle. This increasingly places the responsibility on the clinician to maximize the benefit of ultrasound examinations, while minimizing the risk. Clearly, to make valid judgements, ultrasound users will need to be educated about safety issues. Attitudes that assume inherent safety under all conditions, simply because the equipment is commercially available, should be discouraged. Misplaced assumptions that the highest power always gives the best results need to be replaced by an awareness of the relative risks of each application. Knowledgeable ultrasound technologists will be better prepared to interpret the output display data, and it is the purpose of this chapter to draw attention to some important and relevant issues.

The concept of relying more on an on-screen output display than on output regulation is gaining universal acceptance, although there are some differences between the AIUM/NEMA and the IEC approaches and requirements for manufacturers.

The TI is a quantity that is related to an estimated temperature rise. The longer pulses and higher pulse-repetition rates typically used in pulsed Doppler exposures result in higher average intensities, and therefore involve a greater risk of producing biological effects from heating.

Dwell-time is an important component of thermal dosage because the duration of exposure to ultrasound is directly related to operator skill and examination difficulty. Clearly, acceptable dwell-time is directly related to the level of temperature elevation, in that a higher temperature would be expected to produce biological effects with shorter exposure durations.

The importance of the MI, or similar indicator of risk of mechanical damage, is emphasized by recent research findings. Although there is no direct evidence of adverse effects in humans (no scientifically controlled studies with humans exist) from mechanical bioeffects, the scientific literature contains a considerable amount of information on both *in vitro* and *in vivo* effects in lower animals and mammals. The critical acoustic parameter is pulse pressure and the appropriate dosage expression for cavitation effects is the spatial peak pulse average intensity. Acoustic output measurements reported in Chapter 3 indicate that the peak rarefactional (p_r) pressure amplitudes for Doppler systems range between 0.46 and 4.25 MPa. For imaging systems, the range was 0.66–3.50 MPa. The observation of hemorrhage in the mouse lung following exposure to pulsed ultrasound[2] at 1 MPa has demonstrated that these rarefactional pressure amplitudes are sufficient to lead to adverse biological effects in mammalian tissues.

WFUMB symposia on safety of ultrasound in medicine

The World Federation for Ultrasound in Medicine and Biology has provided substantial resources to sponsor scientific workshop-style meetings of experts from around the world to debate contentious issues on the safety of diagnostic ultrasound. These symposia have resulted in publications that summarize clearly identified topics on ultrasound safety and standardization. The inaugural meeting in Sydney in 1985 demonstrated the need for open international debate and initiated the process of establishing a common forum for dialogue between members of organizations with divergent scientific and political opinions. The primary objective was to formulate scientifically valid recommendations on the safe use of diagnostic ultrasound that may be endorsed by the WFUMB as being a responsible set of guidelines.

In 1988, at the time of the second WFUMB symposium, it was realized that the maximum power output of some commercial equipment was approaching levels that were capable of substantially heating biological tissue. The importance of ultrasound-induced heating has subsequently been fully examined in further workshop meetings, the first of which included 20 invited scientists who were selected on the basis of their contributions to this field of research. The proceedings of the meeting were documented in draft form (WFUMB Working Group, Geneva Report, 1990) and circulated globally for review amongst the scientific and medical community. Copies were sent to each of the affiliated ultrasound societies of the WFUMB. On the basis of this extensive review, a revised document was presented for discussion at a symposium in Hornbaek, Denmark, in 1991. This major meeting was attended by 50 invited delegates including official representatives of the WFUMB, six national ultrasound societies, three standards/regulatory bodies, seven medical ultrasound manufacturers together with individually selected scientists and clinicians. The topic was 'Issues and recommendations regarding thermal mechanisms for biological effects of ultrasound'. The WFUMB has adopted, as official policy, a number of important statements on thermal effects in clinical applications, to cover issues relating to B-mode imaging, pulsed Doppler and transducer heating. The statements are as follows.

WFUMB (1992): Safety of diagnostic ultrasound

B-mode imaging

'Known diagnostic ultrasound equipment as used today for simple B-mode imaging operates at acoustic outputs that are not capable of producing harmful temperature rises. Its use in medicine is therefore not contraindicated on thermal grounds. This includes endoscopic, transvaginal and transcutaneous applications.'

Doppler

'It has been demonstrated in experiments with unperfused tissue that some Doppler diagnostic equipment has the potential to produce biologically significant temperature rises, specifically at bone/soft tissue interfaces. The effects of elevated temperatures may be minimized by keeping the time during which the beam passes through any one point in tissue as short as possible. Where output power can be controlled, the lowest available power level consistent with obtaining the desired diagnostic information should be used.

Although the data on humans are sparse, it is clear from animal studies that exposures resulting in temperatures less than 38.5 °C can be used without reservation on thermal grounds. This includes obstetric applications.'

Transducer heating

'A substantial source of heating may be the transducer itself. Tissue heating from this source is localized to the volume in contact with the transducer.'

During the symposium a number of recommendations were also formulated, and these have been endorsed by WFUMB as being internationally acceptable guidelines for the safety of diagnostic ultrasound with respect to thermal issues.

Following the successful completion of the symposium on thermal effects, the same format was used to examine the subject of non-thermal mechanisms of interaction. Because this topic was rather more diverse than the thermal subject, two intense workshops were conducted over a period of 18 months. The first was held in Utsunomiya, Japan in 1994. The latest *WFUMB Symposium on Safety of Ultrasound in Medicine*, in Germany, 14–19 April 1996, reviewed thermal issues but dealt primarily with non-thermal bioeffects. A number of conclusions were achieved that reflect international consensus. Observers from industry were encouraged to attend, because of the possible implications for the use of echo-contrast media. The proceedings of the symposium have been edited into a comprehensive document[12]. The proceedings of the 1996 symposium have been accepted by the WFUMB executive council. The following is a selection of the clinically appropriate conclusions and recommendations.

WFUMB (1997): Recommendations on thermal effects

'A diagnostic exposure that produces a maximum temperature rise of no more than 1.5 °C above normal physiological levels (37 °C) may be used clinically without reservation on thermal grounds.

A diagnostic exposure that elevates embryonic and fetal *in situ* temperature to 41 °C (4 °C above normal temperature) for 5 min or more should be considered potentially hazardous.'

WFUMB (1997): Conclusions on non-thermal effects

'Capillary bleeding has been observed in the lung after exposure of neonatal, young and adult mice, swine and adult rats, rabbits and monkeys to diagnostically relevant, pulsed ultrasound. Thresholds for capillary bleeding in adult mice and neonatal and young swine are of the order of 1 MPa at 2 MHz, which is within the range of output values of commercially available diagnostic ultrasound systems.

In the air-filled mammalian lung, bleeding from alveolar capillaries has been induced experimentally by ultrasound at diagnostic exposure levels. This effect has not been observed in the fluid-filled mammalian fetal lung. There is no direct evidence to date as to whether or not this effect can occur in humans.'

WFUMB (1997): Recommendations on non-thermal effects

'Currently available animal data indicate that it is prudent to reduce ultrasound exposure of the human postnatal lung to the minimum necessary to obtain the required diagnostic information.'

Contrast agents

'Gas bodies introduced by a contrast agent increase the probability of cavitation. A physician should take this into account when considering the benefit/risk ratio of an examination.'

B-mode imaging

'When tissue/gas interfaces or contrast agents are not present, the use of B-mode imaging need not be withheld because of concern for ultrasound safety. This statement also applies to endoscopic, transvaginal and transcutaneous applications. When tissue/gas interfaces or contrast agents are present, ultrasound exposure levels and duration should be reduced to the minimum necessary to obtain the required diagnostic information.'

Doppler

'When tissue/gas interfaces or contrast agents are not present, and where there is no risk of significant temperature elevation, the use of diagnostic Doppler equipment need not be withheld because of concern for ultrasound safety. When any of the above conditions might be present, ultrasound exposure levels and duration should be reduced to the minimum necessary to obtain the required diagnostic information.'

In addition to these policy guidelines, the WFUMB Safety Committee has published scientific review papers[13,14] to disseminate current information on safety of ultrasound in medicine.

ECURS safety guidelines

The European Committee for Ultrasound Radiation Safety (ECURS) has published a clinical safety statement that addresses the issues of routine use of ultrasound[15]. It states:

'In view of the possibility of ultrasonically-induced biological effects within tissues in the path of a Doppler beam, routine examinations of the developing embryo during the particularly sensitive period of organogenesis using pulsed Doppler devices is considered inadvisable at present.'

This cautionary note was also issued in a guideline for the safe use of Doppler ultrasound for clinical applications[16]; the Committee further advised that:

'Pulsed Doppler exposures become increasingly likely to produce biologically significant local heating as the pregnancy proceeds through second and third trimesters because the acoustic absorption of fetal bone increases with its progressive mineralisation. This is of particular importance when brain or growing epiphyses lie in the path of the pulsed Doppler beam.'

It is important to understand that these statements on clinical ultrasound safety are not regulatory. They provide essential information and serve a useful role in advising users of the potential risk from certain diagnostic ultrasound procedures.

ASUM safety guidelines

The Australasian Society for Ultrasound in Medicine (ASUM) supports the findings of the *WFUMB Symposium on Safety and Standardization in Medical Ultrasound*. In order to encourage the prudent use of ultrasound in clinical examinations the ASUM has endorsed, as official policy, a number of statements on safety issues. Most of the original statements are currently under review, in consideration of important recent research findings, some of which are yet to be published. However, it is unlikely that there will be significant change to the recommendation of prudent use of diagnostic ultrasound in obstetrics. Some relevant extracts of statements follow.

Gray-scale imaging

'Diagnostic ultrasound applied transcutaneously for gray-scale imaging has been in clinical use since the late 1950s. To date the results of numerous follow-up studies on patients and children who had been examined before birth have failed to demonstrate any biological effects that could be attributed to this mode of ultrasonic examination.

Developments in diagnostic ultrasound include the use of endovaginal and endoscopic gray-scale imaging. The safety of these techniques is currently under review. The results to date on patients show no evidence of any harmful effects. However, until more data are obtained, prudent use of these techniques is recommended, i.e. the use of minimum acoustic output and dwell time consistent with that required to obtain the necessary diagnostic information.

Given the known benefits and efficacy of the medical diagnosis, the prudent use of gray-scale imaging far outweighs the risks, if any, that may be present. There is no reason to withhold the application of the technique when it is indicated on clinical grounds.'

Pulsed and color Doppler imaging

'The acoustic output of equipment functioning in the pulsed and color Doppler modes can be higher than that used in gray-scale imaging. Some Doppler equipment has the potential to produce a biologically significant temperature rise, specifically at bone/soft tissue interfaces. In pulsed Doppler the beam is kept stationary and the same tissues are irradiated throughout the examination. In color Doppler the beam is scanned to produce the color image, and the insonation is distributed over a large volume of tissue. For this reason color Doppler produces a lesser effect.

Doppler techniques are used over a range of applications including vascular, cardiac and fetal examinations. Differing maximum acoustic outputs are recommended for these applications. Care should be exercised that the examinations are performed prudently, using as low

as reasonably achievable (ALARA) acoustic output and dwell time.'

In addition to these policy guidelines, the Safety Committee of the ASUM has published scientific review papers[17,18] and newsletter articles to inform the membership and the medical community in general of current issues on safety of ultrasound in medicine.

The ASUM consistently advocates the prudent use of diagnostic ultrasound in medicine. The Society maintains a similar philosophy to that of the American Institute of Ultrasound in Medicine whereby it is considered appropriate to use diagnostic ultrasound when medically indicated, i.e. when there is an expected diagnostic benefit from the procedure. Similarly, the ECURS advises in conclusions and recommendations on transvaginal sonography[19] that:

'The absence of long-term, large scale, follow-up studies following first-trimester ultrasound exposures means that care is required in the application of transvaginal ultrasonography in early pregnancy. It should only be performed for pure medical reasons that are to the benefit of the mother and/or the embryo.'

The tutorial paper also states:

'If the clinician judges it as essential to scan the fetus or embryo with pulsed Doppler or color flow Doppler, the output parameters should be kept as low as possible.'

References

1. AIUM (1991). *Safety Considerations for Diagnostic Ultrasound.* Bioeffects Committee of the American Institute of Ultrasound in Medicine. (Rockville Pike, MD: AIUM Publications)
2. Child, S. Z., Hartman, C. L., Schery, L. A. and Carstensen, E. L. (1990). Lung damage from exposure to pulsed ultrasound. *Ultrasound Med. Biol.,* **16,** 817–25
3. FDA (1985). *510(k) Guide for Measuring and Reporting Acoustic Output of Diagnostic Ultrasound,* 1992 updated Draft document. (Rockville, MD:

Food and Drug Administration, Center for Devices and Radiological Health)
4. Duck, F. A., Starritt, H. C. and Anderson, S. P. (1987). A survey of the acoustic output of ultrasonic Doppler equipment. *Clin. Phys. Physiol. Meas.,* **8,** 39–49
5. AIUM/NEMA (1992). *Standard for Real-Time Display of Thermal and Mechanical Acoustic Output Indices on Diagnostic Ultrasound Equipment.* (Rockville, MD: American Institute of Ultrasound in Medicine)

6. FDA (1993). *Revised 510(k) Diagnostic Ultrasound Guidance for 1993.* (Rockville, MD: Food and Drug Administration, Center for Devices and Radiological Health)

7. Holland, C. K. (1995). Ultrasound bioeffects: the mechanical and thermal indices. In Goldman, L. W. and Fowlkes, J. B. (eds.) *Medical CT and Ultrasound: Current Technology and Applications,* pp. 211–228. (Madison WI: Advanced Medical Publishing)

8. AIUM (1994). *Medical Ultrasound Safety.* (Laurel, MD: American Institute of Ultrasound in Medicine

9. Barnett, S. B. (ed.) (1997). Conclusions and recommendations on thermal and non-thermal mechanisms for biological effects of ultrasound. In *World Federation for Ultrasound in Medicine and Biology Symposium on Safety of Ultrasound in Medicine. Ultrasound Med. Biol.,* special issue, **23**

10. EFSUMB (1996). Tutorial paper: thermal and mechanical indices. European Committee for Ultrasound Radiation Safety. *Eur. J. Ultrasound,* **4**, 145–50

11. IEC 1157 (1992). *Requirement for the Declaration of Acoustic Output of Medical Diagnostic Equipment. Standard 1157.* (Geneva: International Electrotechnical Commission)

12. Barnett, S. B. and Kossoff, G. (eds.) (1992). Issues and recommendations regarding thermal mechanisms for biological effects of ultrasound. In *World Federation for Ultrasound in Medicine and Biology Symposium on Safety and Standardization in Medical Ultrasound. Ultrasound Med. Biol.,* **18**, No. 9, special issue

13. Barnett, S. B., Rott, H. D., Ter Haar, G. R., Ziskin, M. C. and Maeda, K. (1997). The sensitivity of biological tissue to ultrasound. *Ultrasound Med. Biol.,* **23**, 805–12

14. Barnett, S. B., ter Haar, G. R., Ziskin, M. C., Nyborg, W. L., Maeda, K. and Bang, J. (1994). Current status of research on biophysical effects of ultrasound. *Ultrasound Med. Biol.,* **20**, 205–18

15. EFSUMB (1996). European Federation of Societies for Ultrasound in Medicine and Biology, Clinical safety statement for diagnostic ultrasound. Report from the European Committee for Ultrasound Radiation Safety. *Eur. J. Ultrasound,* **3**, 283

16. EFSUMB (1995). European Federation of Societies for Ultrasound in Medicine and Biology, Guidelines for the safe use of Doppler ultrasound for clinical applications. Report from the European Committee for Ultrasound Radiation Safety. *Eur. J. Ultrasound,* **2**, 167–8

17. Barnett, S. B., Kossoff, G. and Edwards, M. J. (1993). International perspectives on safety and standardisation of diagnostic pulsed ultrasound in medicine. *Ultrasound Obstet. Gynecol.,* **3**, 287–94

18. Barnett, S. B., Kossoff, G. and Edwards, M. J. (1994). Is diagnostic ultrasound safe? Current international consensus on the thermal mechanism. *Med. J. Aust.,* 160, 33–7

19. ECURS (1995). European Committee for Ultrasound Radiation Safety, Tutorial paper on Transvaginal ultrasonography – safety aspects. *Eur. J. Ultrasound,* **1**, 355–7

Take-home messages

13

G. Kossoff and S. B. Barnett

INTRODUCTION

The philosophy used by the authors in preparing their chapters has been to provide the reader with a range of selected material that represents important issues and developments in safety of diagnostic ultrasound rather than to compile detailed accounts of publications on the bioeffects of ultrasound. In keeping with that policy, this chapter summarizes key issues, in the form of take-home messages, which are intended to answer some of the commonly asked questions regarding the safety of ultrasound examinations in obstetrics. The European Committee for Ultrasound Radiation Safety has recently published a series of short focused tutorial papers on safety which expand upon some of these messages, and these are referenced in the text. Recommendations by the World Federation of Ultrasound in Medicine and Biology are also included where appropriate for ultrasound examination in obstetrics and gynecology.

ULTRASOUND THERMAL BIOEFFECTS

Does diagnostic ultrasound heat tissue?

Potentially hazardous temperature rises can be obtained in soft tissue. These can range up to 3 °C. Even higher temperature elevation can be obtained in soft tissue near bone, e.g. brain tissue near the skull. Temperature elevations up to 6 °C have been measured in fetal brain tissue at maximum output of current Doppler equipment in studies in which there was little maternal intervening tissue to reduce the fetal exposure.

What affects temperature increase?

While the presence of bone greatly increases the amount of ultrasound-induced heating, vascular perfusion, or blood flow, dissipates some of the temperature rise reached *in vivo*. In highly vascular tissues such as the kidney, perfusion can decrease the temperature by as much as 50%. In brain the degree of reduction is of the order of 10%. Conduction can transfer heat from the point of intersection of the beam to adjacent tissues. Hence, brain soft tissue can be heated by conduction from bone (which strongly absorbs ultrasound) in addition to temperature increase caused by absorption of ultrasound by the brain tissue itself.

How fast does temperature rise?

The rate of ultasound-induced temperature elevation is rapid and a maximum temperature elevation can occur within 1–2 min from onset of the exposure. A biologically significant temperature increase can occur within 30 s of exposure when a fixed beam of pulsed Doppler ultrasound interacts with bone. The effects due to conduction and perfusion become manifest about 30 s following onset of exposure.

Where is the maximum temperature elevation?

Methods have not yet been developed to allow accurate calculation of the position of maximum temperature elevation in tissue. Because of absorption, conduction and perfusion considerations, the position of maximum temperature elevation in soft tissue seldom coincides with the position of maximum axial intensity[1]. If the transmission path is through low-attenuating liquid, such as urine in the maternal bladder, the maximum temperature rise would occur close to the beam focus, perhaps at the fetal skull. However, when the path is through attenuating soft tissue the maximum temperature elevation is obtained quite close to the transducer, typically within a few centimeters.

What about heating from the transducer?

A substantial source of heating may be from the transducer itself[9]. Models used to determine worst-case temperature elevation in tissue do not take into account the effect of transducer self-heating. The resulting temperature rise is limited to tissue close to the transducer; this is important for intracavitary examinations. In external examinations the degree of transducer self-heating is mediated by cooling from the surrounding conditions.

THE RISK OF THERMAL EFFECTS

WFUMB recommendations

The following are excerpts of recommendations by the World Federation of Ultrasound in Medicine and Biology (WFUMB) on thermal effects derived mostly from studies on hyperthermia in animals and from experience in humans[3].

Safe temperature elevation

A diagnostic exposure that produces a maximum *in situ* temperature rise no more than 1.5 °C above physiological levels (37 °C) may be used clinically without reservation on thermal grounds.

Hazardous temperature elevation

A diagnostic exposure that elevates embryonic and fetal *in situ* temperature above 41 °C (4 °C above normal temperature) for 5 min or more should be considered potentially hazardous.

Febrile patients

Care should be taken to avoid unnecessary additional embryonic and fetal risk from ultrasound examination of febrile patients.

Information for users

Users should be provided with worst case estimates of temperature increases for diagnostic systems capable of producing temperature rises greater than 1.5 °C. The risk of adverse effects of heating is increased with the duration of exposure. Safety guidelines should include an appropriate duration factor.

WFUMB policy statement on B-mode imaging[2]

The use of B-mode imaging need not be withheld because of concern for ultrasound safety. This statement applies to transcutaneous, transvaginal and endoscopic applications. This recommendation is based on results of studies which show that B-mode imaging in tissue does not cause temperature elevation greater than 1.5 °C.

WFUMB policy statement on Doppler[2]

It has been demonstrated in experiments with unperfused tissue that some Doppler diagnostic equipment has the potential to produce a biologically significant temperature rise, specifically at bone/soft tissue interfaces. The effects of elevated temperatures may be minimized by keeping the time during which the beam passes through any point in tissue as short as possible. Where the output can be controlled, the lowest available power level consistent with obtaining the desired diagnostic information should be used.

ULTRASOUND NON-THERMAL BIOEFFECTS

This category includes all other bioeffects caused by ultrasound. The two major ones are cavitation-induced effects due to oscillations near naturally occurring or introduced gas cavities and those due to acoustic streaming induced by radiation pressure.

Can cavitation occur in vivo?

It can no longer be stated that diagnostic ultrasound cannot produce acoustic cavitation in the body. There is consistent evidence of cavitation-related bioeffects in animals exposed to pulsed ultrasound at levels achieved by modern diagnostic equipment (see Chapter 7). The effect requires the presence in tissue of gas bodies or tissue/gas interfaces. The clinical implications of these effects is uncertain.

Can cavitation cause tissue damage?

Evidence from animal studies shows that pulmonary and intestinal capillary bleeding can occur at maximum output levels of diagnostic equipment. In the frequency range of 2–10 MHz, the threshold for pulmonary bleeding is approximately 1 MPa, whereas for intestinal bleeding it is approximately 3 MPa.

At present it is not known whether capillary bleeding occurs in humans, or what the long-term clinical implications may be. It is prudent to reduce ultrasound exposure to lungs and intestine, particularly in neonates, who have little overlying tissue. This is relevant to neonatal cardiac examination, in which lung is frequently exposed during a search for a 'cardiac ultrasound window'.

Is there any risk from contrast agents?

Ultrasonic contrast agents and certain procedures such as flushing introduce gas-containing cavities into the body. The presence of these gas cavities increases the likelihood of cavitation and greatly reduces the exposure threshold for initiating cavitationally induced bioeffects. Although no significant adverse health effect has been reported to date, the use of these agents is new and their safety needs to be fully evaluated.

What about acoustic streaming?

Red blood cell and contrast agent stasis, retinochoroidal blanching and body fluid movement in cysts and abscesses are the major bioeffects produced by acoustic streaming induced by radiation pressure. The output of modern equipment is sufficient to produce streaming effects in human liquid-filled organ structures. There is no evidence of hazard associated with this streaming when generated within amniotic fluid or urine in obstetric examinations. Weakly tethered cell structures, and in particular embryonic tissue, could bear the risk of disturbance if the recovery from the application of a transient stress wave is incomplete. Any decision to use diagnostic ultrasound during the first trimester should acknowledge radiation stress as a potential bioeffects mechanism.

Is radiation pressure important?

Recent evidence shows that hemorrhage of fetal tissue in mice[4] can occur at interfaces of bone and soft tissue following exposure to low average intensity pulses emitted by a lithotripter. The effect is not caused by temperature increase. The mechanism is not fully understood, but it seems to be due to impulsive changes in radiation pressure. This is important to obstetrics because the effect has been observed in a range of fetal tissues, with the lowest threshold in the brain.

THE RISK OF NON-THERMAL EFFECTS

WFUMB recommendations[3]

Cavitation

It has been shown experimentally that acoustic cavitation can alter mammalian tissues. It is therefore important to consider its significance in medical applications of ultrasound.

Contrast agents

Gas bodies introduced by a contrast agent increase the probability of cavitation. A physician should take this into account when considering the benefit/risk ratio of an examination.

B-mode imaging/Doppler

When tissue/gas interfaces or contrast agents are present, ultrasound exposure levels and durations should be reduced to the minimum necessary to obtain the required diagnostic information.

ISSUES RELATING TO DIAGNOSTIC EXAMINATIONS

Is fetal growth affected by diagnostic ultrasound?

Multiple examinations of the fetus in the second and third trimesters has been associated with fetal growth retardation in animal and human studies. Studies on fetal growth have suggested the possibility of inducing growth-restrictive mechanisms in various animal models. Growth factors such as insulin-like growth factor and heat shock proteins may be involved in this effect. The results have not yet been independently confirmed.

It is difficult for human studies to confirm a cause-and-effect relationship; they show an association of the effect with ultrasound examinations, but not necessarily the effect of ultrasound itself. Current clinical acceptance of diagnostic ultrasound makes it extremely difficult to set up a definitive study, owing to the need for a large number of matched unexposed controls.

What is the result of epidemiology/human studies?

Some recent human studies have reported an association between ultrasound examinations and low birth weight or increased incidence of left-handedness. It is difficult to prove a cause-and-effect relationship indicating that ultrasound exposure is responsible for the observed effect. The results of epidemiology studies conducted so far indicate that diagnostic ultrasound does not cause major harm to the fetus or to mammalian tissues[5,6]. Our knowledge of the effects of ultrasound scanning on development of the central nervous system remains incomplete.

What is the benefit of routine ultrasound in obstetrics?

The major benefits in terms of pregnancy management stem from early diagnosis of twins and better gestational age determination, both of which may lead to more cost-effective approaches to obstetric intervention. The principal benefits stem from accurate pregnancy dating. The only reasonable benefit to perinatal outcome is the detection of major fetal malformations which leads to pregnancy termination and a subsequent reduction in perinatal mortality. Evidence from randomized, controlled trials of ultrasound at various stages has not shown that routine ultrasound improves pregnancy outcome (Chapter 11).

Spectral and color Doppler examinations

Doppler examinations are performed in two modes. In spectral Doppler the beam is kept stationary and many insonating pulses are used to measure the distribution of velocities in the selected range-gate (all tissues in the line of sight are insonated). In color Doppler (velocity or power) the beam is scanned and only a few stationary insonating pulses are used to obtain the Doppler information. No point in tissue is therefore heated to the same degree.

Should Doppler examination in the first trimester be routine?

In view of a possible bioeffect produced by a Doppler examination and the lack of a identified useful clinical application, it is generally considered inadvisable to perform routine Doppler examination in the first trimester in uncomplicated pregnancy.

The European Committee for Radiation Safety is the only organization to have issued a policy statement on this topic[7,8]. It advises a cautionary approach, suggesting that routine examination of all pregnancies in the early first trimester is not advisable. This is not intended as a regulatory statement, but simply advises prudent use.

Other societies (American Institute of Ultrasound in Medicine, Australasian Society for Ultrasound in Medicine) maintain a prudent policy of using diagnostic ultrasound only when medically indicated, i.e. when there is an expected outcome that will benefit the diagnosis.

Transabdominal vs. transvaginal examinations

In transvaginal examinations the transducer is closer to the tissues being visualized[9]. Thus if the transvaginal transducer was activated by the same energizing pulse as a transabdominal one, the tissues would be subject to greater exposure. Diagnostic systems function in transmitting as well as receiving mode. Being closer to the tissues means that echoes from the tissues are absorbed less during their return to the transducer and a stronger signal is received. Strong transmitting is therefore not necessary and transvaginal transducers are in general not energized as strongly as transabdominal transducers. The net effect is that transabdominal and transvaginal examinations entail about the same order of exposure to the fetus.

How does the mode of operation affect equipment output?

The average intensity depends on the mode of operation. It is lowest for fetal heart monitors, and becomes progressively higher for B-mode imaging, M-mode, Doppler imaging and pulsed Doppler operation, in that order. The average intensity increases for each of the modes listed by approximately a factor of three. There is, however, little difference between the pulse amplitudes used in each of the modes, with the median peak rarefaction pressure a little above 2 MPa for all conditions. The recent relaxation of the regulatory control by the Food and Drug Administration in the USA will result in increases in the mean exposures used internationally, especially in obstetrics.

Are there still any areas of uncertainty?

Despite the many studies that have been undertaken to evaluate the safety of ultrasonic examinations, there are still areas where the scientific knowledge is incomplete. It is known that the central nervous system is sensitive to damage by ultrasound. However, it is not certain that, even if a small lesion were to be produced, the current techniques would be able to identify the effect. Human studies have implicated loss of cerebral lateral dominance (increased incidence of left-handedness) as a possible result of interference with neural cell migration in second- or third-trimester fetuses; however, no ultrasound study has been undertaken to demonstrate such an effect histologically. Most forms of imaging investigations carry some element of risk; imaging examinations are performed on the basis of an appropriate risk/benefit analysis.

MECHANISMS OF INTERACTION

Cell studies

Diagnostic ultrasound is capable of producing a number of bioeffects in cells growing in culture in the laboratory. The implications of these effects on safety is difficult to determine. In particular, the mechanisms of interaction of ultrasound with cells suspended in liquid are not necessarily the same as those that would occur with cells supported in a soft tissue matrix. Whilst these studies are of great benefit to the understanding of mechanisms of interaction under controlled laboratory conditions, it is not certain that the effects noted in cells *in vitro* occur in soft tissue *in vivo*. Therefore, care must be taken in extrapolating results of cell studies to human safety.

Animal studies

Studies on animals provide useful evidence relevant to the safety of the exposure in humans. Interpretation of the results must take into account differences in species and the relative size of the ultrasonic beam. The conclusions of the World Federation of Ultrasound in Medicine and Biology[2,3] on thermal issues were based on hyperthermia studies that used whole-body temperature elevation, where the temperature rise was gradual. With ultrasound the temperature elevation is localized to the size of the ultrasonic beam, and the temperature rise is rapid. The most important recent finding is that of lung capillary bleeding caused by exposure to diagnostic ultrasound equipment. This effect was observed for a wide range of animals, including monkeys. Fortunately, it does not seem to occur in the fetal lungs, where gas is not present.

EDUCATION

Diagnostic ultrasound has the potential for false-positive and false-negative results. Misdiagnosis may be more dangerous than any effect that might result from ultrasound exposure. Diagnostic ultrasound should be performed only by personnel with sufficient training and education.

Significant thermal and non-thermal bioeffects can be produced by exposure to maximum diagnostic acoustic output from modern equipment. It is important that sonologists and sonographers are aware of the substantial changes to acoustic output that can occur when the settings of the equipment are altered during examinations[10]. A better understanding would be achieved from knowledge of exposimetry, including ways to measure acoustic output[11] and the non-linear effects of distortions in the acoustic waveform that can occur during propagation[12].

High-power modern ultrasound equipment can incorporate a display, in real time, of the thermal and mechanical index[13]. This is described in Chapters 7 and 12. This form of output display is intended to give the user an estimate of the relative risk of producing thermal or cavitation-related bioeffects. The indices are designed deliberately to have no defined quantity but, simply, to indicate the likelihood of causing an effect. Hence a higher value for TI or MI represents a greater risk and the user should consider reducing the duration of exposure and the need for the examination.

Users of ultrasound are encouraged to adopt the ALARA principle (as low as reasonably achievable); routine use of this principle is a matter of good practice[14].

References

1. NCRP (1992). *Exposure Criteria for Medical Diagnostic Ultrasound: 1. Criteria Based on Thermal Mechanisms*. Report no. 113. (Bethesda, MD: National Council for Radiation Protection and Measurements)
2. Barnett, S. B. and Kossoff, G. (eds.) (1992). Issues and recommendations regarding thermal mechanisms for biological effects of ultrasound. *World Federation for Ultrasound in Medicine and Biology Symposium on Safety and Standardisation in Medical Ultrasound. Ultrasound Med. Biol.*, **18**, special issue
3. Barnett, S. B. (ed.) (1997). Conclusions and recommendations on thermal and non-thermal mechanisms for biological effects of ultrasound. *World Federation for Ultrasound in Medicine and Biology Symposium on Safety of Ultrasound in Medicine. Ultrasound Med. Biol.*, special issue, in press
4. Dalecki, D., Child, S. Z., Raeman, C. H., Penney, D. P., Mayer, R., Cox, C. and Carstensen, E. L. (1997). Thresholds for fetal hemorrhages produced by a piezoelectric lithotripter. *Ultrasound Med. Biol.*, **23**, 287–97
5. European Committee for Radiation Safety (1994). Tutorial paper: Diagnostic ultrasound: genetic aspects. *Eur. J. Ultrasound*, **1**, 91–2
6. European Committee for Radiation Safety (1996). EFSUMB tutorial paper: epidemiology of diagnostic ultrasound exposure during human pregnancy. *Eur. J. Ultrasound*, **4**, 69–72
7. European Committee for Radiation Safety (1995). EFSUMB: Clinical safety statement 1994. *Eur. J. Ultrasound*, **2**, 77
8. European Committee for Radiation Safety (1996). EFSUMB: Clinical safety statement for diagnostic ultrasound (1995). *Eur. J. Ultrasound*, **3**, 283
9. European Committee for Radiation Safety (1994). Tutorial paper: Transvaginal ultrasonography. *Eur. J. Ultrasound*, **1**, 355–7
10. European Committee for Radiation Safety (1995). EFSUMB: Ultrasound radiation safety tutorial: What happens when you alter the settings on your diagnostic ultrasound machine? – safety considerations. *Eur. J. Ultrasound*, **2**, 229–30

11. European Committee for Radiation Safety (1994). Tutorial paper: Principles and methods of field measurements. *Eur. J. Ultrasound*, **1**, 279–82

12. European Committee for Radiation Safety (1994). Tutorial paper: Non-linearity and finite amplitude effects. *Eur. J. Ultrasound*, **1**, 213–15

13. European Committee for Radiation Safety (1996). EFSUMB: Tutorial paper: thermal and mechanical indices. *Eur. J. Ultrasound*, **4**, 145–50

14. European Committee for Radiation Safety (1995). EFSUMB: Guidelines for the safe use of Doppler ultrasound for clinical applications. *Eur. J. Ultrasound*, **2**, 167–8

Index

absorption coefficient, variation between tissues, 27
acoustic output,
  control of, 69
  measurements of, 15, 16, 17
  variations in between ultrasound techniques, 15
acoustic power,
  conventional transducers, 16
  Doppler mode, 17
  endovaginal transducers, 17
  output, 10, 69
  values in diagnostic ultrasound, 16, 17
acoustic pressure cf. radiation pressure, 88
acoustic streaming, 87, 135
  definition, 90
  effects in obstetrics, 95
  effects on soft tissue, 95
  in biological materials, 91
  in diagnostic ultrasound exposure, 91
  in limited spaces, 92
  in vivo, 92
  in water, 91
  internal stresses on tissue and, 94
  neurosensory responses to, 96
  non-linear propagation effects of, 92
Aerosomes®, 74
AF0150®, 75
Albunex®, 78, 80
  clinical studies, 81
American Institute of Ultrasound in Medicine (AIUM),
  Bioeffects Committee, 122
  model on temperature elevation in diagnostic ultrasound by, 28
  model on temperature elevation in first trimester, 29
  on-screen labelling of output display standards, 123
amplitude,
  comparison between modes of operation, 18
  measurement of, 16

animal studies,
  fetal growth after ultrasound exposure, 40
    mechanisms for, 41
    murine, 240
    simian, 240
  fetal hematopoiesis, 43
  fetal neural response to ultrasound exposure in sheep, 56
  hyperthermia in mice and rats, 27
  interaction mechanisms, 137
  myelination in lamb, 45
  myelination in rat, 45
  temperature elevation and bone marrow cell
  proliferation abnormalities, 33, 34
  temperature elevation and rat embryonic development, 33
  temperature elevation in fetal guinea-pig brain, 31
attenuation, 4
Australasian Society for Ultrasound in Medicine, safety guidelines, 129

B-mode imaging,
  changes in since 1970, 20
  exposure levels in cf. M-mode, 16, 17
  International Guidelines on Safety with regard to Thermal Issues WFUMB Recommendations, 36
  safety guidelines, 127
  spatial peak temporal average intensity levels in, 18
  WFUMB policy statement on, 134
  WFUMB recommendations on, 128, 136
beamwidth, 4
benefit vs. risk, 99
  research methodologies, 99
bioeffects,
  non-thermal, 134
  of contrast agents, 76
  of hyperthermia, 133
  thermal, 133
birth weight, ultrasound exposure and, 102

bone, measurements of temperature increase
    in, 30
bone marrow,
    proliferation abnormalities after
        temperature elevation exposure, 33,
        34
Bubbicles®, 75

cancer, ultrasound exposure and, 109
Cavisomcs®, 80
cavitation,
    animal models of, 63
    bubble contrast agents and, 79
    chromosomal damage by, 55
    collapse of cavitation nuclei, 65
    echo-contrast agents and, 67
    energy limits and, 13
    evidence *in vivo*, 65
    hemorrhage in lung and intestine and, 66
    hydrodynamic, 73
    in fetal lung, 55
    inertial,
        definition of, 64
        mechanism of, 64
        prediction of, 64
    mechanism and effect of, 55
    occurrence of, 135
    potential for *in vivo*, 67
    risk indicators, 67
    WFUMB recommendations on, 135
cell membrane effects, 55
childhood cancer, ultrasound exposure and,
    109
chromosomal damage by cavitation, 55
clinical significance of sensitivity to ultrasound
    exposure, 59
congenital malformations,
    cardiovascular, 101
    ultrasound exposure and, 100
contrast agents,
    bioeffects, 76
    free bubble, 74
    gas bubble, 74
    history of, 73
    in biological media, 78
    in cell-free media, 78
    lipid-encapsulated bubble, 74
    medical applications of, 75
    microbubble, 74

non-vascular applications, 75
    response of bubbles to ultrasound, 76
    risk from, 135
    safety of, 76
    WFUMB recommendations on, 128, 135
cost–benefit analysis, 118
cost-effectiveness,
    cost–benefit analysis, 118
    first-trimester ultrasound, 114
    frequent obstetric ultrasound
        examinations, 118
    placentography, 117
    RADIUS trial, 117
    routine Doppler in pregnancy, 116
    routine obstetric ultrasound, 113
    second-trimester ultrasound, 114
    small-for-gestational age fetus scanning,
        116
    third-trimester ultrasound, 116
cytokines,
    response to temperature elevation, 42
    role in fetal growth, 42

decibel notation, 7
diagnostic ultrasound,
    current impressions on safety, 39
    fetal effects of, 136
    frequency of use, 39
diagnostic ultrasound vs. therapeutic, 22
Doppler,
    ASUM safety guidelines on, 130
    color, exposure from, 17
    continuous wave, exposure from, 17
    cost-effectiveness of routine obstetric
        scans, 116
    exposure levels from attachments to
        scanning equipment, 19
    International Guidelines on Safety with
        regard to Thermal Issues WFUMB
        Recommendations, 36
    operating intensities, 19
    pulsed,
        changes in since 1970, 21
        exposure from, 17
    safety guidelines, 127
    use in first trimester, 136
    WFUMB policy statement on, 134
    WFUMB recommendations on, 129, 136
dwell-time, safety guidelines, 126

echo-contrast agents, *see under* contrast agents
EchoGen®, 75
Echovist®, 74
    clinical studies, 81
education,
    importance of, 138
    vs. regulation, 121
embryonic development, effects of
    temperature elevation on, 32
encapsulated microbubble contrast agents, 74
endovaginal transducers, exposure levels cf.
    conventional probes, 17
equipment Output Display Standards, 123, 124
European Committee for Ultrasound
    Radiation, 125
    safety guidelines, 129
exencephaly, after temperature elevation *in
    utero* in rats, 33
exposure,
    acoustic power output, 10
    and birth weight, 102
    and congenital malformations, 100
    and fetal growth, 102
    and malignancy, 109
    and neurological development, 106
    and neurosensory development, 106
    comparison of levels measured in
        free-field, 19
    control of by operator, 23
    diagnostic vs. therapeutic, 22
    fetal growth after, 40
    free-field cf. *in situ*, 16
    increase in since, 1970 20
    limits on and cavitation considerations, 13
    limits on and thermal considerations, 12
    measurement in water cf. *in situ*, 12
    measures of from conventional
        transducers, 16
    measures of from Doppler mode
        ultrasound, 17
    measures of from endovaginal
        transducers, 17
    multiple, 110
    parameters used to describe, 9
    peak negative pressure, 12
    reliability of measurements of, 19
    spatial peak pulse average intensity, 11
    spatial peak temporal average intensity, 10
    trends in, 20

FDA,
    acoustic output limits set by, 123
    model used by in prediction of *in situ*
        exposure from free-field
        measurements, 16
    relaxation of controls by, 1, 15
febrile patients, 134
fetal activity, as a response to ultrasound, 56
fetal brain, response to ultrasound, 44
fetal growth,
    effect of diagnostic ultrasound on, 136
    in vivo studies, 40
    mechanisms for changes, 41
    retardation of, 60
    role of insulin-like growth factor axis in, 41
    ultrasound exposure and, 102
fetal heart monitors, intensities used by, 19
fetal hematopoiesis,
    in vivo studies of, 43
    mechanisms for, 44
    ontogeny of, 43
fetal intestine, hemorrhage in, 66
fetal lung,
    cavitation effects in, 55
    hemorrhage in, 66
    lesions in after ultrasound exposure, 46
    radiation pressure as a cause of lesions, 47
fetus,
    temperature elevation,
        in fetal head, 30
        in second- and third-trimester fetus,
            29
Filmix®, 74
first-trimester model of temperature elevation,
    29
first-trimester ultrasound, cost-effectiveness,
    114
fracture repair by ultrasound, 56
free bubble contrast agents, 74
free-field exposure cf. *in situ*, 16
    FDA model for prediction, 16
FS069®, 75

gas bubble contrast agents, 74
gray-scale imaging, ASUM safety guidelines
    on, 129
growth, *see under* fetal growth
growth factors, temperature elevation and, 41
guidelines,

international, 125
safety, 126

heat shock proteins,
    role in fetal growth, 42
    temperature elevation and, 41
    thermotolerance, 42
heating, *see under* hyperthermia
Helsinki Ultrasound Trial, 104
hematopoiesis,
    fetal,
        in vivo studies of, 43
        ontogeny of, 43
    mechanisms for, 44
    simian, 43
hyperthermia,
    bioeffects of, 133
    biological effects of, 32
        thresholds of, 32
    clinical significance, 33
    clinical significance of, 59
    conduction of heat in tissues, 28
    effect on cytokines, 42
    effect on growth factors, 41
    effect on heat shock proteins, 41
    estimates of ultrasound-induced
        temperature increases, 28
    gross effects of, 35
    international guidelines on safety, 36
    risk estimates, 35
    risk of, 134
    risk of and imaging method used, 27
    teratogenic effects of, 35
    teratogenic effect thresholds, 27
    tissue responses to, 57
    transducer heating and, 36
hysterosalpingography, 76

indocyanine, 73
insulin-like growth factor, role of axis in fetal
    growth, 41
insulin-like growth factor binding proteins, 41
intensity,
    definition of, 6
    distribution of, 7
    measurement set-up, 11
    spatial peak pulse average, 11
    spatial peak temporal average, 7, 8, 10

interaction mechanisms, 137
interleukins, 42
International Guidelines on Safety with regard
    to Thermal Issues WFUMB
    Recommendations, 36
international standards and guidelines, 125

left-handedness, after ultrasound exposure, 56
Levovist®, 74, 79
    clinical studies, 81
lithotripsy,
    cf. diagnostic ultrasound, 22
    power used for and bioeffects of, 66
lung, fetal, 46, 55, 66
lung hemorrhage, 60
lung lesions after ultrasound exposure, 46

M-mode imaging,
    changes in since 1970, 20, 21
    exposure levels in cf. B-mode, 16, 17
malignancy, ultrasound exposure and, 109
mechanical index,
    Output Display Standards for, 124
    safety guidelines, 126
microbubble contrast agents, 74
microphthalmia, after temperature elevation
    in utero in mice, 33
monitoring systems, cf. other systems, 19
MRX115®, 74
myelination,
    development in fetus, 45
    ex utero studies in rat, 45
    in utero studies in lamb, 45
    in utero studies in rodents, 46

National Council for Radiation Protection
    and Measurement (NCRP),
    model on temperature elevation in
        diagnostic ultrasound by, 28
    model on temperature elevation in first
        trimester, 29
National Electrical Manufacturers Association
    (NEMA), model on temperature elevation
    in diagnostic ultrasound by, 28
    on-screen labelling of output display
        standards, 123
neural response by fetus to ultrasound, 56
neurodevelopment, 45

neurogenesis, fetal, 45
neurological development, ultrasound
    exposure and, 106
neurosensory development, ultrasound
    exposure and, 106
neurosensory responses, to acoustic
    streaming, 96
non-thermal sensitivity, 54
    cavitation, 55
    cell membrane effects, 55
    neural response, 56
    streaming, 56

operator, need to understand exposure
    control, 23
organogenesis, congenital malformations and
    ultrasound exposure, 100
Output Display Standards, 123, 124

peak negative pressure, 12
peak rarefaction pressure, 16
    in pulsed modes, 18
    increase in since 1970, 20
    values in diagnostic ultrasound, 16, 17
physiotherapy, exposure levels used in cf.
    diagnostic levels of time averaged
    intensity, 22
placentography, cost-effectiveness of routine
    obstetric scans, 117
power, definition of, 6
propagation of ultrasonic waves,
    mode, 3
    velocity, 4
pulse pressure, safety guidelines, 126
pulsed mode of operation, 5

radiation force, definition, 88
radiation pressure, 135
    cf. acoustic pressure, 88
    definition, 88
    gradient, 89
    profile, 88
radiation stresses, 87
    in diagnostic beams, 88
    in pulsed vs. continuous waves, 89
    radiation force, 88
    radiation pressure, 88, 89
RADIUS Study, 104, 117
regulation,

success of, 121
    vs. education, 121
risk,
    vs. benefit, 99
        in routine first-trimester scans, 122
        research methodologies, 99
risk indicators for cavitation, 67
routine obstetric ultrasound examination,
    benefit, 136
    cost-effectiveness of, 113
    Doppler, 116
    first trimester, 114
    frequent, 118
    placentography, 117
    RADIUS trial, 117
    second trimester, 114
    small-for-gestational age fetus, 116
    third trimester, 116

safety committees, 121
safety guidelines, 68, 126
second-trimester ultrasound,
    cost-effectiveness, 114
sensitivity, clinical significance of, 59
sensitivity to ultrasound,
    non-thermal, 54
    variations in, 53
SH U 454®, 74
SH U 508A®, 74
small-for-gestational age fetus, ultrasound
    cost-effectiveness for, 116
soft tissue,
    acoustic streaming effects on, 95
    measurements of temperature increase in,
        29
soft tissue model of temperature elevation, 29
spatial peak pulse average intensity, 11, 16
    values in diagnostic ultrasound, 16, 17
spatial peak temporal average intensity, 7, 8,
    10
    average values, 15
    in B-mode imaging, 18
    increase in since 1970, 21
    Output Display Standards for, 124
    values in diagnostic ultrasound, 16, 17
speech development delay, after ultrasound
    exposure, 56
standards, international, 125
streaming, ultrasound-induced, 56

temperature elevation,
  acoustic energy limits and, 12
  bioeffects of, 133
  biological effects of, 32
    thresholds of, 32
  clinical significance, 33, 59
  effect on cytokines, 42
  effect on growth factors, 41
  effect on heat shock proteins, 41
  estimates of ultrasound-induced, 28
  first-trimester model by AIUM, 29
  first-trimester model by NCRP, 29
  gross effects of, 35
  in second- and third-trimester fetus, 29
  international guidelines on safety, 36
  maximum, 133
  measurements of ultrasound-induced *in
    vitro*,
    bone, 30
    soft tissue, 29
    tissue-mimicking phantoms, 30
  measurements of ultrasound-induced *in
    vivo*, fetal head, 30
  risk estimates, 35
  risk of, 134
  see also hyperthermia
  soft tissue model of, 29
  teratogenic effects of, 35
  tissue responses to, 57
  transducer heating and, 36
  use in physiotherapy, 22
teratogenic efffects, of hyperthermia, 27
therapeutic ultrasound, cf. diagnostic, 22
thermal index,
  display of during equipment operation, 28
  Output Display Standards for, 124
  safety guidelines, 126
thermal sensitivity, tissue variation in, 57
third-trimester ultrasound, cost-effectiveness,
  116
tissue heating, 133
tissue repair by ultrasound, 56
tissue-mimicking phantoms, 30
tissue/gas interfaces, 68
transabdominal vs. transvaginal, 137
transducer,
  exposure levels from conventional, 16
  exposure levels from endovaginal, 17
transducer heating, 36, 35, 134

transducer heating, safety guidelines, 128
tumor necrosis factor-α, 42

ultrasound,
  changes in since 1970, 20
  comparison of exposure levels, 16
  comparison of modes of operation, 18
  diagnostic vs. therapeutic, 22
  hyperthermia and imaging method used,
    27
  operators' need to understand exposure
    control, 23
  properties of ultrasonic waves,
    attenuation, 4
    beamwidth, 4
    decibel notation, 7
    intensity, 6
    mode of propagation, 3
    non-linear, 6
    power, 6
    pulsed mode, 5
    velocity of propagation, 4
    wavelength, 4
  radiation stresses in pulsed vs. continuous,
    89
  response of bubble contrast agents to, 76
  tissue repair and, 56
ultrasound exposure, *see under* exposure
ultrasound-induced heating, *see under*
  hyperthermia
ultrasound-induced streamimg, 56
Ultravue®, 74
urinary reflux, 76

velocity of propagation, 4

wavelength, definition of, 4
World Federation for Ultrasound in Medicine
  and Biology (WFUMB),
  clinical safety conclusions, 68
  conclusions on non-thermal effects, 128
  development of, 123
  International Guidelines on Safety with
    regard to Thermal Issues, 36
  policy statement on B-mode imaging, 134
  policy statement on Doppler, 134
  recommendations, 58, 128
  recommendations on B-mode imaging,
    136

recommendations on cavitation, 135
recommendations on contrast agents, 80,
    135
recommendations on Doppler, 136

recommendations on temperature
    elevation, 134
safety guidelines, 127
tissue/gas interface conclusion, 68